# The Untold Secrets Of Permanent Weight Loss

## *(Deception in the American Diet Industry)*

by

## Jim Cabeceiras

Bloomington, IN 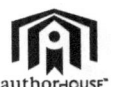 Milton Keynes, UK

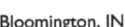

*AuthorHouse™*
*1663 Liberty Drive, Suite 200*
*Bloomington, IN 47403*
*www.authorhouse.com*
*Phone: 1-800-839-8640*

*AuthorHouse™ UK Ltd.*
*500 Avebury Boulevard*
*Central Milton Keynes, MK9 2BE*
*www.authorhouse.co.uk*
*Phone: 08001974150*

*First published by AuthorHouse 6/26/2006*

*ISBN: 1-4259-4042-0 (sc)*

*Printed in the United States of America*
*Bloomington, Indiana*

*This book is printed on acid-free paper.*

*Credits: Adriana C. Photography of Hammond, Louisiana, Ponchatoula Fitness Center of Ponchatoula, Louisiana.*

# Preface

If your health is the single most important commodity you own, why then, do most of us eat too much, live a substandard quality of life, and die before our time? Are you willing to spend the last twenty years of your life as a semi-invalid ? After all, many Americans are doing that now. Think about what's in store for us in the future with the national crisis we face now. Think about your future. There a many questions you need the answers to, but first you need to be educated enough to know what to ask. You will discover many new principles and guidelines as you read on. Guidelines that, though they are valid and essential to your personal success, are not widely accepted and often 'hidden away' by the diet industry. Why? Simply put, it's a path of least resistance where the objective is to make as much money with as little effort as possible. Understand that I am not a mouthpiece for corporate America. I have no hidden agenda. I am just one man who questions the powers that be, understands and practices the principles that are valid, and wants to enlighten you. Your decision to adopt and practice these guidelines is entirely up to you.

With all the disingenuous hype and propaganda that's out there, there is still an upside to what appears to be a dark cloud on the horizon. The good news is that, despite the fact that you and I will always be irrational and impulsive in our thought processes, the solution to permanent weight loss allows you to be yourself, with all your emotional flaws, and still lose the weight you desire to lose. What I provide for you here is a way out of the chaotic world you exist in now. With all the misguided information and influences that seem to point to a better life for you, understand that there is only one genuine pathway to your personal success.

Let's start with the exposure of the truth. The truth about our culture, our nature, and the valid principles and guidelines that, if applied, will lead you to your own promise land. Losing weight has never been and never will be just a process of food selection. Virtually every diet in America will fail to give you any lasting results because nutritional advice is only ten percent of your problem. What you will discover as you read on will be your salvation from the other ninety percent of your challenge, or, in simple terms, what it takes to take the weight off and keep it off. At this moment in time, we are indeed facing a national health crisis with our rate of obesity and the number of Americans that are considered overweight. Many of us are so desperate, we seek salvation by worshiping the false prophets of our time - weight loss centers, fad diets, surgery, harmful stimulants, or even prescription drugs. Believe that our collective desperation and ignorance is part of this dangerous mix. The deceit dished out by the diet industry and other so-called experts complete this spectrum of smoke and mirrors. What are the results? In most cases, it's continuous failure and frustration. You may or may not be one of these people. You may have had moderate success in the past. Either way, the discovery process I offer you now will help you gain perspective and accomplish your goals.

We live in a country that offers many freedoms. Free will is one of them, but most of us fall short of realizing and living the best life we can, and we only have ourselves to blame. I offer you a choice now. Continue on the same path of moderate and temporary success where you put your faith in what 'they' tell you. Continue to live in constant anguish and inner conflict because your will power is constantly tested and you always seem to lose that inner struggle. Or, you can empower yourself by gaining the knowledge you need to become leaner, healthier, happier, and more energetic than you ever thought possible. It's your move.

# Table of Contents

## Chapter 1
### Our Diet Culture - Propaganda and Myth Exposed

It is common knowledge that, in America today, the effort to 'diet' is as popular as its ever been throughout our history. We all know friends and family members who have restricted their meals and lived in misery for the time they were disciplined enough to control their impulse to over-eat. 'Diet' has become a negative word in our culture. With all the books, tapes, infomercials, and general media overload on the subject, why, as an entire nation, are we collectively frustrated? Why are so many Americans overweight? Why did your last attempt to lose weight become only temporary? After all, you started your diet with great expectations of success, and though it seemed to work in the short run, it just didn't work for you as time went on. Sound familiar? It's only natural to feel dazed and confused with the choices you are confronted with. As America approaches levels of obesity never seen before by man, there is desperation in the air, my friend, and desperation is bad. If you are desperate (be honest here), you are primed and ready for a magic carpet ride. Desperation has caused despair throughout our history, where the masses simply follow an ill-fated leader, and the few end up taking advantage of the many. The street word for it is "scam". Some diet concepts are scams. Simply a clever attempt to prey on yours and anyone else's desperation. Some diet plans mean well, but they still don't offer any real solution. Not for you. In fact, when you think about all the specialized diets we have to choose from today, do any of them offer anything other than groceries, ideas on what groceries are best, or deal with any concept other than 'what to eat'? I challenge you with this question now because I want you to begin to understand our free market and it's effect on all of us. As you read on, you will come to an understanding about our culture, why diets fail again and again, and the impact on all of us who blindly follow these 'experts'.

Beware of the choices you have in America. I had a friend who spent $79.00 a week on his "special food", as he attempted to shed some winter fat on a diet plan that offers its own groceries. Keep in mind the $79.00 was for him only! Scam? I'll let you be the judge. So let me pose a question to you. Are diets bad for us? Is there a common flaw in most diets that doom them to failure in your case? The answers are "no" and "yes". For many people, and maybe you fit in here, diets are a temporary effort to drop a few pounds (or many pounds), and they can be, and often are, mildly successful. The problem is, no matter how effective a diet is, it rarely addresses the source of your problem, which, in all cases, is related to how your 'inner voice' and your engrained habits control your appetite, and impulses that influence your choices of foods. Most diet philosophies and formulas deal with the physical - your body's response to changes in habits and foods. What to eat and when to eat it. That's why they fall short of solving your issues of weight management. It's the primary reason we all struggle with the latest and greatest diet. Our instinctive drives for food, shelter, love, sex, and comfort are driven by very primal resources in our brains, and unless you can understand and alter the way you deal with these primal drives and their lifetime effect on your behavior, you are doomed to only nominal success, and, more often than not, only temporary success in your effort to shed pounds. Think about the generic approach diet experts and corporations use in books, videos, and commercials. Do they know what your specific challenges are? Does the 'one diet fits all' approach really work? Hell no! It's easy and irresponsible to market a mechanical 'Here's a list of what to eat and how much' diet. Understand that most diet books on the market today have sound nutritional advice, but they leave out vital information and advice that apply to you. Specifically, your efforts to gain control of your impulses, understand your history of flawed thinking, and overcome years of poor habits. You are left on your own with a list of groceries, when to eat them, and how much to eat. One percent of your problem is solved! Oh, boy! What progress! This media myth will be explored further as you read on.

As I mentioned earlier, there are many false prophets out there feeding on the desperation of the masses. That is just another common denominator of our nature. Our basic instinct to 'follow the crowd' is at play here, too. Poor habits and influences originate from both your environment and your mind. Every human being who, at this moment in time, is overweight, has a specific set of 'flawed rationales' for eating too much or too often. If you are severely overweight, you should seek counseling so that the source of your behavior can be discovered and steps can be taken to help you alter your attitude towards nutrition. Your flawed, irrational thinking will sabotage any diet you choose to begin, especially if you have a food addiction or an emotional problem that needs to be addressed. What are the negative motivators that distort our thinking and cause many of us to eat for reasons other than what nature intended? Will your habits automatically change when you start on the next diet? What makes dieting such a destructive cycle of failure after failure? The answers are simple. **The type and quantity of food you eat is far less important than your rationale for over-eating.** More importantly, how do you find your own set of faulty motivations and take steps to correct them? Keep this in mind as you read and you will discover the truth behind the cloak of corporate and media hype that have been feeding you their grocery list of propaganda.

### Common Myths

If you live in America you have probably been pounded by cultural rhetoric and media driven dog and pony shows. Our culture is now controlled by common ideas and philosophies that are adopted by the majority, and therefore must be right for everyone. Wrong. At this point in time, most of what is pushed on us by the majority, such as new, improved concepts in diet and exercise, are suspect. The worst thing you can do as an individual is sell out to the concept that you must own an SUV, watch 2.5 hours of television each day, rent movies the critics tell you are good, and listen to music that you think everyone else likes so you are not viewed as a ' strange, rebellious one'. I tell you these things because media and cultural influence in America is as strong as ever. Yet, obesity in America is also at its pinnacle, so what is happening to us? Well, in a nutshell, you, as an individual, need to stop buying what they are selling, and really start thinking for yourself. This really takes discipline. Are you up to the task?

As part of the deprogramming you must go through to become permanently lean, the myths involving your own culture and attitudes have to be in question regarding nutrition. Let's explore a few of these more harmful 'accepted common truths'.

**Fasting - It's a fast, effective method for weight loss.** Maybe for a bear in hibernation or an alligator after swallowing a gazelle, but for us humans, not eating for an entire day is bad news. It may be a spiritual endeavor for some, or just the simplistic declaration that 'hey, if I don't eat at all, I'll lose more weight'. But it's bad. Why? In short, food is actually a catalyst for losing weight. Now that I have you a little confused, let me explain. Think of your body as an engine that burns hot at times and cold at times, but never shuts off. Two major forces influence the speed, or rate of burn of your engine. Voluntary activity, such as physical exercise, and the involuntary activity that occurs within your body. We call this activity your metabolism. Metabolism involves every involuntary function of your body, such as your heartbeat, breathing, brain activity, digestive processes, organ functions, maintenance of your core body temperature, and the continuing process of everything at the cellular level that result in heat, or the burning of calories. Think of metabolism as your 'engine'. Your body, even at 300 pounds, is in need of constant, daily fuel, and to starve yourself will always have negative consequences. Not eating for two days will probably not stop your heart, but it will slow your metabolism down to a crawl, and with your engine at a very low idle, your fuel (calorie) requirements are even less than before. Oops! Backfire! Fact is, timing is just as important as the food itself. If you could eat six small meals a day instead of three larger ones, your metabolism would burn hot, even without much exercise. Change a few of the foods you eat and you burn even hotter (more calories per day). So this is good news, right? Now you can eat every day, and all day if you so desire. Sure you can and should, but within reason. If fasting is, in fact, something that you practice spiritually from time to time, be sure to drink plenty of water or other nutritional fluids. You should now have a clear understanding about the negative influences of starvation. Believe it or not, there are many educated people that think the one meal a day plan works for them. So if you are a 'faster' or just 'not into breakfast', get over yourself and accept what I tell you at face value. The fact is, depriving your self of food for long periods leads to overwhelming cravings for rich and fatty foods, or, even worse, the potential to become a binge eater. It's just bad for you. Your body is reacting to your own self-induced starvation by craving and storing more fat than ever before! Yikes! Let's move on.

**Carbohydrates are bad.** Why, until just recently in America, did carbohydrates become evil? Could carbohydrates be the scapegoat for our problem of obesity in this country? Let's examine this. As a people, we have consumed potatoes, rice, bread, and pasta for hundreds of years. In 1930, the average American was nowhere near 30 pounds overweight. The same is true up to the 1950's, so as a nation with a weight problem in 2006, how did we make that leap of logic to find carbohydrates as a culprit? Allow me to explain. The fault lies with the development of our culture over the past fifty years. We are the laziest, most undisciplined people in the world, and we are on slippery slope traveling downhill at record speed. Sure, diets promoting the consumption of meats (protein), with little or no 'carbs' have been successful, but has anyone ever done this throughout a lifetime? How about fifteen years? What are the results? The fact is, little is known about diets that promote one food group over another. But I can tell you what we do know. The steak, bacon, eggs, pork, burgers, and the cheese you consume on a 'high protein low carbohydrate diet' contain high amounts of saturated fats. These are fats that are bad for you. Really bad. Bad for your heart and arteries is just a beginning. Remember what I said before. The millions of people who follow this diet do not justify its success, which is short term at best. Even the masses can be ignorant and temporarily fooled, and this is definitely the case here. In addition, whether you accept it or not, your body was designed for balance - meaning protein, carbohydrates, and yes, even some fats. Let's look at the 'body as an engine' analogy I used earlier. Carbohydrates are fuel for your engine, with simple carbohydrates (sugars) providing the quick source of fuel, and complex carbohydrates(whole grains, rice, vegetables, oatmeal, etc.) for long, sustained energy. The problem we have with obesity now has no correlation with the evil carbohydrate. We just consume the wrong types, we consume them in mass quantities, and we exercise very little. These 'trash' carbs are found in soft drinks, processed sugars, or anything that's been refined to the point where it has virtually no nutritional value. In fact, if everyone in America were to eliminate 'trash carbohydrates' from their diet, our national weight crisis would probably dissipate within six months. It's just a theory, but I challenge anyone to dispute it. Understand that the best sources of carbohydrates are natural, non-processed foods. Fruit juices, natural honey, and other 'fructose' sources are the best simple carbohydrates. Natural complex sources should also be part of your daily diet. 'Carbs' provide energy that your body constantly requires and offer a wide array of nutritional benefits. They are a perfect compliment to a well -rounded diet, but you should limit their consumption. Take the time to reflect on your own attitude about carbohydrates and the skewed message you get from the diet industry. Bottom line, the experts are not going to appear in a commercial and insult you because you've been sitting on your ass. The easy approach to separating you from your money is simply to push any diet that eliminates or severely restricts your carbohydrate consumption. You get to sit on your ass, the diet corporations keep their stockholders happy, and you fall into the trap of always looking externally for answers. Understand that your rationale of 'helplessness' is dangerous and self- defeating. Accept the concept of 'carbs' as an energy source. Accept the fact that your poor exercise and nutritional habits are the problem here. Accept all this as truth, and you can begin to reverse your cycle of frustration. Remember, if you require more fuel (a five- mile hike), then you can and should consume more carbohydrates. If you require less fuel (watching someone walk five miles), you need less. It's not rocket science! Refer back to the underlying theme of balance, and you will understand that carbohydrates are not fallen angels from purgatory.

**The curse of the slow metabolism.** This is a dangerous, self-rationalizing 'story' many of us invent. The bigger problem is the distortion of what is the accepted truth today. Most Americans are completely ignorant of their own biology, and this rationale is dangerous. Your metabolic rate is not completely out of your control. For the sake of simplicity, let's define metabolism as the rate of burn, or the pace at which your body burns calories. You here terms such as 'base metabolic rate' used in the personal trainer's world, but what you really should be aware of is that your personal rate, or pace of burning calories, is not set in stone, and can be increased through alterations diet, exercise, changes in lifestyle, and even changes in the levels of your anxiety or stress. At this moment, you should know or have some knowledge of how many calories you burn daily. If you don't, I suggest you buy a calorie counter and monitor your intake and weight for a few weeks. You can increase your calorie burn rate by simply changing the times you eat. Six small meals per day keeps your furnace burning hot, while three large meals only keep you in 'lukewarm' status. Raw, wholesome grains and fibrous foods such as oatmeal or raw vegetables increase your metabolic rate by increasing the workload of your digestive system. A raw carrot, for example, is bulky, fibrous, and low in calories relative to size and weight. It takes more calories for your body to process and break down a carrot than it would, say, a brownie of equal weight. Exercise is a no- brainer. Move around more, burn more calories. Activity creates heat, and heat increases the rate of your calorie burn. Understand? In addition, if you packed on a few pounds of muscle, your 'base rate' or daily burn rate would also increase. Muscle cells require more nourishment and effort on your body's part to maintain than fat cells, therefore, two people can be the same age, height, weight, ethnicity, and even have the same eating habits, yet have totally different rates of burning calories if one has added five pounds of muscle while the other has added five pounds of fat. Even a subtle change in the number of hours you sleep will alter your metabolism. It makes sense. Heart rate, breathing, and other functions slow down when you are inactive. I'm not suggesting that your metabolism can be altered dramatically. What I am telling you is that you can influence your own natural processes in small increments by changes in diet and exercise. Yes, your metabolism slows with age, but your challenge is to overcome this 'built in' excuse for weight gain that allows you to rationalize the fact that you will never be your former self. I just want you to be keenly aware of this influence so you can eliminate any history of flawed beliefs that you may have accepted as truth over the years.

So, what have we learned here. Well, for starters, metabolism is not a curse you are born with. Granted, there are cases of medical conditions that may or may not contribute to obesity, but these conditions are rare. Not being in control is the lie we tell ourselves to justify failure. That's just human nature at work. If anyone ever uses the 'I have a slow metabolism' rationale in my presence, there will be hell to pay. Hey, if I won't lie to you, why should I let you lie to yourself. Am I making any sense here?

**To be successful with your diet, you must eat 'recommended' foods.** A true statement, but only a partially true statement that fails to acknowledge the fact that not all of us our complete masters of our domain. Your diet will be successful if you regulate your 'cheating', not eliminate it. Why? Because you and I do not have the powers to deny our nature, our culture, or years of engrained habits. That's why. The misconception involves the elimination of you and your habits, desires, and attitudes about food. Your diet can and will be successful, even with some indulgences, but the reason for failure has nothing to do with 'cheating'. Constant cheating is a by-product of a habit of behavior that, if not altered, will always lead to failure. Again, your ability to regulate your 'cheating' is the fundamental reason for avoiding failure, not the fact that you failed to follow a specific, recommended diet. Understand? As I said before, most diets are considered temporary solutions to a lifetime discipline. After all, a diet, by today's standard, means restricting and possibly altering your food intake. But if you are thirty years old, and you decide to follow a diet (consume less calories) to drop a few pounds, what are you really trying to accomplish with your attitude toward food? By eating well balanced, healthy meals in smaller quantities, we all mean well in the beginning. But then what happens? You eventually go back to your old habits of eating. What the hell! You lost the 10 pounds so the diet was a success, right? Oh so wrong, my friend. As a thirty something adult, you have at least twenty -five years of cultural, family, and behavioral influences on your attitudes towards food. Let's say, for the purpose of this example, you dieted for two months to lose the ten pounds you desired. How can you expect to reverse twenty- five years of influence and engrained behavior in just two months? The answer is you can't. This uphill battle, for most of us, puts us in a position where the only result is failure. This hidden challenge leads me to the next shattered belief you should be aware of.

**Your past - A denial by the 'Experts'.** In addition to mental processes that differ from person to person, there is failure by the industry in general to acknowledge your specific history of weight gain. Why is this relevant? Well, before anyone can make any claim about product or philosophy on weight loss, your past has to become the foundation, or starting point, for beginning to break your cycle of failure. Let me explain just how critical your history is. Your rate of descent is predetermined by your own rate of ascent. If, for example, you find yourself forty pounds overweight after ten years of gradual gains, your healthy rate of weight loss will be slow and gradual, and it may take several months or more, not weeks or days, to reach your ideal weight. Understand that your challenge becomes more difficult because weight gained over several years involves almost permanently engrained habits, flawed or irrational thinking, lack of impulse control, and other factors that contribute to your status now. More time is obviously needed on your part to correct your 'path' and de-program. You may have experienced a less difficult form of this challenge with, for example, weight gained over the holiday season. Ten pounds gained over 60 days can literally be taken off in a few weeks without much sacrifice or mental de-programming. During your developmental teenage years you may have been lean and active, but if your gains came slowly over the next ten or twenty years, it's still going to be a challenge. If you were overweight and possibly inactive during your teenage years, you may need some form of counseling or psychiatric help to break through a lifetime of emotional barriers and poor habits. Remember, moving forward, that the philosophy of fast-on, fast-off, is valid, but weight gained slowly over the years needs to be managed with a long term effort. You should understand now how ridiculous any claim of weight loss would be by any company or individual without knowing your personal history. The next time you see an article titled 'Lose ten pounds in Ten Days', you can translate the real message: 'You people are idiots - Now buy a subscription you pathetic, dependent sheep'. It's a little over the top, but it makes you begin to think and learn the difference between the truth and the deceit that many Americans fall prey to. Let's move on.

**Food consumed in the evening will be converted to fat.** In most cases, the common belief here is that this conversion occurs the very next day! I could never figure out the origin of this legend, but I can tell you I've heard it thousands of times. Let me set you straight. Bottom line, it's not that late night bowl of ice cream that's packing on the pounds, it's the fact that your daily diet consists of more calories than you burn in a day. It's that simple. In fact, if you are exercising on a regular basis, especially with weights, it may help you to ingest some protein and carbohydrates later in the evening. Keep in mind that your eight hours of sleep is the longest period of time you spend without eating. If you ate nothing from seven p.m. to seven a.m., you have now extended your starvation period another four hours! Let's remember the engine again. A snack or two in the evening helps to keep your calorie burn in the moderate to high range, and as long as your not eating chips and ice cream in large quantities every night of the week, you should be just fine. Remember this moving forward. Excess calories are converted to fat, but the process is an accumulated effect. It takes days (not one night), for an overload of calories to show up as body fat. If you doubt me, consult a nutritionist or a local personal trainer. Hopefully, in your mind, this perpetuated myth has now been laid to rest.

**'I lost 20 pounds on the Super-Trim-Loss Diet Plan.'** Simply put, this is the common myth of what I call 'false credit'. Most companies and authors try to blow this one by you, and you don't realize just how much your intelligence has been insulted. If I told you to eat 1,500 calories a day and you will drop 15 pounds in 6 weeks, what have I done? I basically gave you the roadmap. That's all. Unless your diet is seriously out of balance (Twinkies for breakfast, lunch, and dinner), then the source of your calories is really a secondary issue. After all, you are in fact on your own, dealing with your cravings, attempting to overcome past habits, and visualizing your own possible outcome. The point I make here is that of responsibility. No diet plan, no marketing entity, and certainly no individual can claim credit for your own personal success. If you lose twenty pounds by eating specific foods or supplements, the fact remains that it was you in control of the process 99.9 percent of the time. It was your discipline. Your sacrifice. There is no third party to take credit for what you accomplish through your own efforts of self-control and self-sacrifice. These companies disguise the truth in their advertising and thousands of false claims are made every day at your expense. Here's a typical advertisement: "Wendy lost fifteen pounds and two dress sizes on the super- trim-loss plan - and in just three weeks! You can too! Call now!" Sound familiar? Wendy lost fifteen pounds because she made a conscious decision to sacrifice. She had to manage her own demons and create her own rationale for 'why' she needed to lose fifteen pounds. More often than not, a dramatic reversal by anyone on the road to obesity is typically 'event driven' or 'desire driven', where the motivation to restrict food intake becomes greater than the need to over-eat. Understand? There are hundreds of motivating factors for losing weight, and when Wendy finally reached this breakeven point, whatever diet plan she chose to follow becomes just a by-product of her conscious goal. She had to manage her own time, especially the time in between her meals, where there is no roadmap to follow. The Super-trim-loss people sold her groceries. Even a twenty minute counseling session twice a week does not justify any credit to anyone other than Wendy. The fault here lies with the reasoning that outside forces control our actions most of the time. Truth is, you, and you alone, are in control of much more than you think, and I will uncover more universal truths about human behavior as you read on. The most despicable part of the false representations is the reason behind them. It's your desperation and desire to believe the new and different that's at the core of their motivation, and, as I mentioned before, their first responsibility is to make a profit. No laws are broken. It's just a simple case of unethical deception on the masses by the few. Let's explore this a little deeper.

We know that our natural response to hunger is to eat. But then, many of us do not stop there. Remember what I said about the 'why we eat' being more important than 'what we eat'. Unless you are willing to address the issue of 'why', every diet you attempt will be a constant struggle. Diet products, self- help books, and those break-through fat- burning pills are pounded into your head through constant repetition in the media. The issue they fail to address is that of your individual make-up and the flawed rationale that is yours alone to manage. But they will take your thirty dollars for a month's supply of 'super fat burners'. Understand that this angers me and you should be aware and dissatisfied too. As a consumer, you are a dollar sign. Nothing more. They (The Diet Propagandists) rely on constant consumption on your part. The last thing they want you to know is that dieting will be successful without the consistent use of 'special foods or recommended supplements'. What they want from you is continuous consumption. However, in the real world, taking a day or two off each week may benefit you by eliminating the cravings you may have that seem to dominate your emotional state from time to time. Keep in mind that you and I are flawed and will always be flawed in our thinking processes. It's not a bad thing. It's a human thing. None of us need to suffer, however. The attainment of discipline over irrational desires and negative emotional states will empower you and give you a great sense of well being, but it will never take place twenty four-seven. Look at every claim by every diet company with a suspicious eye, especially if they market their own 'food' or supplements. Remember that throughout the history of modern man, millions of people have lost weight without the use of diet products. Makes you wonder about the past twenty years. Fact is, we are almost in a state of national crisis now with our rate of obesity, yet we have more diet 'breakthroughs', diet products, and appetite suppressants than ever before. What happened? The answer lies again, in our collective willingness to worship false prophets, our collective complacency, and the soft, politically correct direction our culture has taken recently. If I designed a diet that would allow the consumption of cake, ice cream, pizza, and cookies, advertised it as the diet that let's you cheat every day, chances are I would become a millionaire in the blink of an eye. I wouldn't be able to sleep at night, but I would be a wealthy man.

**In essence, we are all told that rather than work to correct our weaknesses, it's o.k. to rationalize our state of 'false dependency', live in a state of denial, and give up control to outside influences.** The message is, 'No effort is needed - we welcome all that want to remain flawed and lazy. We do so love your money'. You need to accept this not as sarcasm, but as reality. Believe me when I tell you that your environment is meaningless relative to your thought processes. We all tend to rationalize our inability to control impulses and what we feel are emotional flaws. To be even mildly successful in losing weight, you have to first admit the fact that you lie to yourself hundreds of times each and every day. We all do. The difference between success and failure is an understanding of the conscious role you play in dealing with the universal tendency to escape from the real world. Reality, in its purest form, is harsh and unacceptable to most of us. It's human nature to rationalize your thinking. We all feel the need to 'escape' to some degree. You and I have a built-in, defiant nature when it comes to facing the real world, all day, every day. It keeps us sane. The key to your success, not just in dieting, is recognizing and understanding your instinct to defy the truth. The 'bad inner voice' we all have that tells us that something or someone else is always to blame, or, in many cases, that eating for pleasure is acceptable in our culture because everyone does it all the time. In the make-up of our Psyche, we all have a built in resistance to things that are good and bad. Believe me, resisting the need to 'conform' or believe in outrageous claims is a good thing. Looking outside yourself for immediate and permanent solutions will doom you to a life of frustration and despair, and, yes, that is a very bad thing.

## Chapter 2

### Damn you, Fast Food

Excuse the language, but I'm trying to make a point here. Many of the pitfalls we face as a common culture is our need to excuse our own discipline (or lack thereof). This may be a tough pill to swallow, but swallow it you must. After all, we are all in control of what we put in our mouths. Free will is a beautiful thing, but without discipline, a deadly thing. In defense of society, the obese man who files a lawsuit against a fast food chain because their cheeseburgers gave him multiple health problems, is justified and righteous, huh!? After all, this poor man is bombarded with hours of fast food commercials, billboards, and a restaurant at practically every corner. He grew up in an environment where he had no choice. So reward him millions as the 'blame game' destroys modern civilization. Remember the slippery slope? We are moving a little faster now. The point I am making here is that of control. Though we all find reasons to consume food that may have nothing to do with real nutrition or fuel needs (remember the engine), we all have to deal with negative motivators. What are these motivators that cause us to veer into the drive through for cheeseburgers and fries? There are many, and most of us have a few of these in combination working against us.

## Deprogramming and Discipline

Remember the primary reason behind the failure of most diets? I talked about the 'why' being more important than the 'what'. Years of influence, good and bad, have already occurred in your life. Your personality has developed. You are now who you are. Your identity is as diverse as a fingerprint, so as an individual, you have your own set of motivations for eating more than you really need to, or making poor choices in nutrition. Your family attitudes have spilled over, and cultural influences are having a go at you, too. One more reason why your last diet failed. **Diets fail to acknowledge negative motivators that relate to you personally**. Most diets in America today, be they published or on videos, market only the easy, mechanical approach to food and health. The 'what'.

"Eat the food we recommend and you will be lean and healthy forever". But don't fret, my friend, I can still help you if you are willing to take a close, hard look at yourself. Let's start a journey of self-discovery.

I have good news for you. Food is good. Food is great. It's the computer inside your head that's been malfunctioning over the years. Most people live their entire life without understanding the simple motivators that affect us all. What are they? First, let's begin with the good.

## The 'Why' Factor

Let's examine the core of your psychological make-up. The layman's answer to the question of 'why' we eat is naturally related to hunger. Of course. Your body is in constant need of fuel, and it is relentless in its demand. No new information here. But is hunger positive? Shouldn't we try to invent a pill that will block hunger? Man, that would be sweet! The answer is yes. Not to the pill invention, but to the positive effect of hunger. It's our biology. Why fight it. Let's say for the sake of example that you, in fact, are perfect. No flaws. You never have a negative thought, never feel stress, and have never been influenced by your environment. Now that you are indeed an android (human robot), your only motivation for eating is fuel and nutritional support.

It's that simple. You need a balance of meats, grains, fruits, vegetables, etc. to maintain a healthy, lean body, so you focus on nutrition for health and look at food as a fuel source for energy. There it is! Problem solved. We can all go home now. Not so fast, my food-obsessed friend. The problem here is that you are an emotional, illogical, rationalizing human being (yes, you are). So your desire for nutrition and fuel have been tainted, just like everyone else in our modern culture. Besides, eating is by no means a mechanical response to hunger. Emotions play a role because your sense of taste and smell play a role, and in the spectrum of our senses, eating can be a very dominant form of pleasure. It's that simple. We know what is positive, but how can we begin to explore the negative? And more importantly, where do you fit in? Let's begin, as a famous Yogi would say, at the beginning.

In our fast-paced, quick-fix modern world, we are an all consuming, spoiled nation of drones. Like pathetic sheep to the slaughter, we are slaves to what the world tells us to bow down to. Most of us, anyway. Your own attitudes toward eating are influenced from childhood, and this 'attitude' you have about food is usually a little skewed as you mature into adulthood. Your cultural, social, and family influences have more than likely led you astray, and I can assume this with confidence, because, after all, you are reading this book. This bad imaging is the single most destructive influence on you or anyone else. Six course meals for dinner, fried chicken on Sunday, family gatherings that center around large, tasty meals and snacks, and the years of an improper way of thinking have taken its toll on America. If you can't change your outlook on food, and I am not saying it will be easy, but if you won't accept that your thinking is defective, I can't help you.

Let's take a closer look at modern man. What happens when availability of food is no longer a problem. Certainly, in centuries past, without electricity and modern commerce, we had limited availability. A daily hunt for meat, maybe a five -mile hike to find berries and nuts (I'm not exaggerating here). Food was fuel. Food was nutrition. People were leaner, too. Attitudes were different. Go figure. So what happened? Well, now we have two problems. First, food is everywhere. Few people are starving in this country. So why would constant availability of food be a problem? It isn't on its own. Add to this mix a collective lack of personal discipline, cultural and media influence, and the limited knowledge most of us have, and there you have it. Gasoline on the fire, so to speak.

Discipline(or lack thereof) and attitudes toward food are at the base, and, therefore, the cause, of most of your attempts to control your weight. But let's dig deeper. What are some of the sub-texts to your way of thinking causing this sabotage. There are reasons you eat that are not related to real nutritional needs at all. Boredom, Anxiety, depression, comfort, self-esteem issues, and, in general, the stress of living your life influence your desire for food and your ability to control negative centers of influence. Let's not forget the outside sabotaging sources, such as social and cultural expectations (peer pressure), and the urge we all have to behave like everyone else. Like a fingerprint, your motivations for over-eating are uniquely yours and yours alone to manage (Again, information intentionally kept from you). Your quest is to determine what drives you to the other side, where nutrition and fuel are no longer primary motivators. Unless you can address the source of your conflict, you will always be a slave to your own demons. You may need to seek counseling if you suffer chronically from anxiety, depression, or other form of mental disorder, especially if it radically influences your diet. Don't play the blame game. It isn't the local burger barn's fault that you are overweight. Listen intensely to your inner voice and understand your flaws. Stop living in a state of defiant ignorance. You alone are in control. There is no excuse for you not to understand the basics of diet and nutrition, unless you don't want to, and in that case, you have a built-in excuse to fail. I've heard people many people claim; "Man, I wish I had more discipline. I just can't seem to stick to a diet. Oh well, that's me." Give me a break. Only a coward takes on the philosophy of 'If I never try, I will never fail'. It's the perfect, self-rationalizing statement that originates from self-loathing and cowardice. It's time to move on.

## *Chapter 3*

### The Path To Your Own Discipline

Examples of our impulsive, rationalizing weaknesses are everywhere. I have come to the realization, and you will too, that it is almost expected of us as a culture. What's wrong collectively with America is simply a collective lack of discipline. In our attempt to become a utopian society where nobody gets hurt emotionally and an 'air of deception' by the powers that be seems to be the status quo, most of us have become mentally and physically weak. We are, in fact, encouraged by our culture to become complacent. Let me explain. Life is not supposed to be a cakewalk. Life is competitive and challenging, especially if you decide to excel at something, and painting our civilization with pretty colors and not acknowledging our nature as a people is a big mistake. It's the challenges of life that make each of us strong as individuals. For your own intellectual growth, challenges are a necessity. Children should be disciplined and taught the value of nutrition and exercise at an early age, but teachers and parents don't want to be too hard on them. Hey, here's a novel idea. Let's not even keep score at little Jimmy's little league game. That way, the losing team doesn't get their feelings hurt. Let's cut down on strenuous exercise at recess and in other activities, and, while we are at it, maybe serve fast food in the lunchroom at school. Don't want to make the kids unhappy. Hey, wait a minute.... we are already doing these things! Oops! I don't offer this analogy just to be callous. I offer this as a warning to everyone as to the direction our culture is taking. The spoiled child has parents running in circles. Literally. In our society, we keep looking for new ways to keep our children content, rather than force them to become disciplined, well behaved, and responsible. How does this analogy relate? Easily. We are now a nation of grown up spoiled people, used to the good life, which, in America, means almost no moderation on anything, good or bad. Discipline is on the decline and so is healthy nutrition and exercise. What are most Americans doing about it? They are looking for outside help through personal trainers, coaches, weight loss clinics, surgeons, drugs, and diets that promise unbelievable results with almost no effort or self control on our part. We now wear our shirts outside our pants like it's a fashion statement (talk about collective denial), and rationalize our thinking so we never have to look in the mirror and see what is really there. If everyone around you is twenty pounds overweight, then it must not be such a bad thing, right? Is there any incentive to become 'the strange, rebellious and disciplined one' in the eyes of society? Valid questions, indeed. Are you beginning to understand how soft and politically correct our culture has become? Do you understand that this is a dangerous direction? Do you understand, too, that the human condition cannot be softened, or our culture will be doomed? We should all acknowledge our nature, embrace it, and never run away from this reality. After all, in today's atmosphere of never inflicting emotional distress on others, I am labeled as 'the bad guy' if I will not allow you to think of yourself as slim when you are not. How confrontational! How dare I!? In 1960, a weight loss clinic was a virtual unknown. Now, there like Starbucks, and just as expensive! Today, you are part of the majority if you packed on twenty pounds as an adult. There is no incentive, at least externally, for you do take action or begin to take control of your diet and health. Again, your defective thinking allows you to rationalize that you are like most everyone else, and that is just fine. I'll explain later why this 'need to fit in' rationale can be a roadblock to your personal success. As a culture, we have collectively weakened our resolve, and I for one, refuse to take part in this irrational, politically correct way of living. Now, take a look at your own attitude. Chances are, if you are overweight and struggling to lose the pounds you've gained over the years, some of your thoughts are self-defeating too. If you cannot inherit the belief that, as an adult, you are truly in command of your thoughts and actions, you are doomed to misery and frustration. Accept the fact that it is 'just you' now and above all, resist the temptation, at all costs, to blindly follow. If you are still blaming someone or something else for your diet and exercise challenges, get over it.

Becoming more self- disciplined is difficult. Resisting the temptation to fit in, to please others, to gain acceptance, and to venture into unknown territory is even more difficult. I admit all this to you. It's a challenge, with the illogical, emotional brain most of us have, to stay the course. Results, because they involve conscious attempts to improve the way you think and manage your impulses, are hard to measure. But you can get help. Books on eastern philosophy, yoga, martial arts, or a valid attempt on your part to learn the art of meditation can have very positive results. Seek and you shall find. I call it development of the 'loner' mentality. Somewhere along the way you must question authority (the diet industry), think for yourself, and resist the temptation to become a sheep in the herd. You do this by investing in yourself. Work deliberately on exercising and strengthening your mind. Take the initiative to educate yourself. You will discover that being in control can be very empowering, and empowerment itself will be a distraction from your own faulty reasoning.

You may be asking yourself how all this rhetoric relates to you personally. Truth is, whether it applies or not, the first step towards any kind of discipline in your life is your own ability to identify your flaws. The identification and acceptance of your flaws gives you a starting point on your journey. You cannot move forward without some form of clarity of these irrational thought processes. When you boil it all down, you, and only you, are responsible for your thoughts and actions as an adult. The blame game has to end here and now.

## Control Issues

Part of your mental mastery, if you are to be even marginally successful with permanent weight loss, lies in the depths of your flawed thoughts and how to go about correcting them. Now, let's look at control and how you apply it to yourself.

Look at each day as a division of two worlds, because we all live in two separate dimensions. We are faced with two issues each day. What we can control and what we cannot. Plain and simple. Your attitude, your speech, your reactions, your physical appearance, and, yes, even what you eat are under the domain of your control. The opinions of others, the weather, the media, and how many fast food commercials you see in one day cannot be controlled. If you eat partly because of stress, chances are your stress is needlessly self-imposed. You may be trying to control people or things you cannot influence, or worse, not admitting to yourself that your state of mind is ultimately yours to control. In the course of your daily life, when things occur, good or bad, how much do they effect your attitude? Understand that this shift of blame to outside forces is the single most irrational lie most of us deal with. It's such a heavy burden to admit this, but if you cannot, you will be doomed to only mediocrity in everything you do in life. This includes your effort to lose weight.

If you think you cannot eat properly because of your job or not having the time, you are lying to yourself. Remember, all of us, including you, seem to always find the time to do the things we really want to do. This applies to exercise, too. You are in control if you take the initiative. Understand that many people who over-eat do so because of self-induced emotional stress. Having a 'bad day' or dealing with bad news are just two of the triggers that send many of us to the comfort of food, even when we feel no real hunger. Am I striking a nerve here? Here's a flawed inner voice you may be able to identify with: ' Look what they made me do! If I wasn't so stressed out, I could be more in control of my diet'. A common, but dangerous mistake we all make in our effort to deal with stress is the irrational, but comforting decision to blame others for the way we feel. Understand that if you spend your life feeling as though you are at the mercy of your environment, you are doomed to mediocrity. The biggest internal lie most of us deal with is the rationale of a 'helpless existence', where anything but the truth tends to dominate your thinking. You have two choices. You can take control by accepting the blame, or you can continue to respond to the rest of the world as if you are helpless and at the mercy of others. Take the high road, here. There can be great liberation and enlightenment for those who control their emotional state most of the time.

Now that you understand control, you can take steps to gain more control over your own impulses and state of mind.    I'm not suggesting a never philosophy of hard-core beliefs that junk food and restaurants are bad. After all, some foods taste really good, and we should allow ourselves some indulgence every now and then. Here's where I fall back to my philosophy of balance. You are human.  You should let yourself go sometimes. You are inevitably going to give in at some point in time during the course of your diet efforts, so why not control it?  Being impulsive every now and then is fine, if done in moderation.    Remember, weight loss is a relatively short- term discipline.  Once you have reached your goal, the long term discipline of maintenance and balance kicks in, and if you still have control issues, even though you are successful in losing weight, staying lean and healthy from that point forward will be too much of a challenge.  Your denial of what can be controlled will always lead to frustration and failure.  Get on board this train, where you take ownership of your health. The empowerment alone will raise your confidence into the stratosphere, and you can deal with any challenge. If you are in control, you can use that fourth of July barbecue as a day you eat for pleasure, and let yourself go.  Be realistic with yourself, set goals of fat loss that are reasonable, and most of all, do not be impatient!

## Are You a Master or a Slave?

There are many control issues that often navigate our conscious mind. If no man (or woman) is an island, then we are all influenced, in some form, by our environment and other people. For some, the need to be loved, accepted, acknowledged, or held in esteem by others is an overwhelming drive. How strong is your desire to conform? The human need to conform, or be 'in agreement' with the majority, can be quite strong. If you feel this need, or feel pressure to accommodate the rest of the world, you, my friend, are truly going to have issues with control. If your strings are being pulled externally (outside your own center of influence and judgment), you, in fact, are a slave. What I am telling you here is that you have no control over others, so why would the opinions and behaviors of other people be important to you? Especially if your conclusion or solution to weight loss seems to be in conflict with these opinions and behaviors. Your 'character' as a person is defined by how you view yourself, not by the opinions of others. Keep in mind that most people are slaves and are unaware of their dependency on 'impulse control' and their built-in necessity to follow someone else's lead. As a master, your impulses are under control and managed to a level that far exceeds the normal. For example, do you reciprocate in kind or 'react' to others socially, or take charge of your own emotional state most of the time. We all have impulses that must be managed. Understand that as an adult, impulse control is a learned behavior skill that evolved from your childhood. Without it, you would more than likely end up in an institution or prison. After all, we have all had the impulse to 'smack someone around', but few of us take it to the extreme. This is good news in that you now know you can improve on the level of your own control. Your first step in this effort is already completed because you are now aware. You must look at your own lack of impulse control as a weakness that can be strengthened over time with some effort on your part. Again, diet companies and even respected authors of diet books often fail to disclose the fact that without impulse control, 'what' you eat becomes meaningless. The good news here is that total change is not necessary. In many cases, only minor alterations in your faulty reasoning are needed to set you on the right path. Many people believe that a 'complete overhaul' of their eating habits and impulses are the only answer, and that flawed thinking is setting you up for failure too. Forget about going from one extreme to the other. Again, it conflicts with the philosophy of balance, and leads to emotional disorders such as bulimia and binge eating. Now, take a look-see into your own world and begin to make subtle changes in your thinking. Believe me, the sacrifice and effort of just a few months will put you on the path that leads from slave to master.

Although it is difficult to deal with emotionally, you must become your own master. Forget about what others think of you or how you are perceived by the world. You don't need the stress and self-doubt baggage that comes with the slave's life. Resist the urge to blindly follow. How can you stay the course with your diet and exercise goals if you are constantly giving in to the influence (pressure) of others? Especially when most of the people you know are poor centers of influence! You cannot. To cross the bridge from slave to master is not easy. It can be lonely. Some people may begin to dislike you for the simple, often subconscious reason that they find you too independent or abnormal. If you often find your friends and loved ones calling you 'stubborn' or 'headstrong', chances are you have a strong sense of self and will accomplish most of what you set out to do. Keep in mind that most people are followers and not independent thinkers. This one cultural situation alone is responsible for the collective laziness in our society. After all, if a million people use a common approach to dieting, it must be the right thing to do. Right? The point I make here is that the majority can be wrong, and in this case, they are. Take, for example, the concept

41

of what a 'meal' is in our country. Most of us have an understanding that large, one thousand calorie meals are normal and even worse, necessary. Restaurants 'super-size' our meals to accommodate the 'big meal' habit of eating. It's done by millions of people every day, but it's bad and it's destructive. This means that the majority of Americans are wrong in their approach to eating! Are you beginning to understand the need to question and become steadfast in your convictions? It's easy to join the millions of people who think that infomercials, drugs, weight loss centers, surgery, and fad diets are the answer.

## Role Models

To be successful in losing weight permanently, you must come to another important understanding. **Role models are few and far between.** If the majority of your family and friends are normal, well- adjusted people, it will be rare that you can find anyone to emulate. Very few people in your world are worthy of emulating. After all, and I can say this with confidence, most of us were raised in a typical fashion, with poor to average perceptions of proper nutrition and exercise. If your mom and dad were tri-athletes, with degrees in nutrition, never allowing you to experience the pleasure of a bowl of Sugar Frosted Toasties, Lasagna, or just a lazy weekend, absent of all exercise, then, yes, you have a strong foundation and a model to follow. But the fact is, most of us don't because these freaks of nature are rare. We call them 'health nuts' because their behavior and habits are so abnormal compared to the status quo. If you can identify with friends and family members who fit this description, then do so. But do not depend on them to take the lead. The initiative to take action and create and implement a valid plan has to come from you. Be happy and welcome any support that comes your way, but do not expect it.

The pressure you feel to fit in and to follow without question is a strong influence, especially when we are young. In modern times, we have the added pressure to conform to a general population that is collectively overweight. Now, you must deal with the emotional stress of isolation, as well as your own internal resistance to change. I tell you this because, if you know what to expect, you will fear this change a little less. Are you beginning to understand the need to develop a 'loner mentality' when it comes to your nutritional and exercise habits? Even if your personality is extroverted, or people oriented, you can still conquer this challenge. First, you come to the understanding that your isolation plays only a minor role in your everyday life. It's not as big a sacrifice as you might think when you break it down in increments of time. Then, you begin to identify with any true role model you can, though there may not be many to emulate. You must accept the fact that going against the grain may seem fruitless, but in the end, after you cross the bridge from slave to master, it will be rewarding. You will always be content when control is yours to own and many of the stresses you felt before are gone. So move forward and stop being the slave that you have been to the rest of the world. Don't let society, culture, or the attitudes and beliefs of others dictate your thinking, especially when it comes to your nutrition. Your success depends on it. Not only in your success in dieting, but for your ability to meet and conquer all the challenges in your life.

## Your Irrational, Frustrating World (How to Escape From It)

Many diet books today, and some of the articles in popular magazines talk about 'quickie' diets designed to shed those ten pounds for the ultimate summer figure. Right? You've read them. Is it healthy to lose ten pounds in one week? Probably not. But you are desperate, so you buy into it. It's your defective thinking at play again. You are in control of what you eat most of the time, and if you find yourself as a dinner guest, you are still in control of the quantity you eat. No matter how busy you are, you still have time to eat right most of the time. If you think otherwise, then you simply cheat yourself with your own irrational thoughts. You escape from this buffer of lies that surround you by becoming a realist. More precisely, that inner voice we all have has to migrate from the idealistic 'dream world' to the harsh world of reality and a recognition of real human behavior at work. You must look inward for answers. Your flawed thinking is the direct result of living in worlds where you convince yourself you have no control. This may be a tough challenge, but there is no book or philosophy or super-duper diet plan that will deliver you from your defective thinking. You must work directly on your own attitudes. We all eat more than we should for many reasons. You may simply love the taste of food. Anxiety could be a motivator for you. In most cases, before you can begin to work on yourself as an ongoing project, you may have to make some major, sometimes temporarily painful changes, and morph into a new you. There is something behind your condition, and you must find what that is. It is not going to be easy. Eating in America can be very pleasurable. Desire for good cuisine can be a very strong motivator. It has to be channeled and controlled. And something has to take its place.

## Substitution Therapy

As an emotional, often irrational human being, you and I are subject to the laws of human nature. When a desire is not fulfilled, whether it be food, sex, love, shelter, or acceptance, there is a void that becomes vulnerable to outside influences. Denying yourself of tasty treats and fine dining creates a stress that has to be dealt with. Diet books and diets in general (the experts) fail in their attempts to disclose this condition because they offer nothing in replacement of your desire to eat for reasons other than to provide nutrition and fuel. Why? Because the 'true' approach to permanent results is more detailed, more involved, and much too challenging for our impatient culture. 'They', meaning diet experts, corporations, authors of diet books and publications, simply tell you want you want to hear. Supply and demand at work, Right? Ah, the almighty dollar.

So how do you fill this void as you begin your diet? Simply put, **you must find an alternative passion. One pleasure must be substituted for another.** It could be a hobby or a project (like writing a book), or a more pleasurable and exciting love life, sex life, a variety of interests or activities, or even the pursuit of dreams and desires that are not related to your sense of taste. Get the picture? Other than that cheeseburger you had for dinner, what really makes you content? What puts you in a frame of mind where food is a craving far removed from your thought process? This type of substitution therapy is a must if you want long term success. Each and every week you have a hundred hours to deal with - to manage cravings, to deny impulses, to think about your next culinary moment of pleasure. This 'void' is the part of your daily life that becomes overwhelming unless you can navigate your thoughts into other areas. **The single largest myth in the dieting world is the fact that very few diet companies or 'Experts' in the media focus on the psychology of managing your time between meals. Remember this fact as you read on because your long -term success depends on how your own time is managed.** If you currently view food as anything but nutrition with the occasional pleasure, your attitude is flawed and you do have a void that will have to be addressed. The issue of impulse control is at play here, too. Remember, it's not complete control that you are after, just more than you have now. De-programming years of habit can and will be difficult. Of all the senses we have - taste, sight, sound, smell, or feeling, taste is a true delight, and to deprive yourself of one sense will mean that others will play more dominant roles. Understand that your enjoyment of eating needs to move way down the scale. In fact, if it will help, make a 'top ten' list of the things you enjoy. If food is anywhere on your list, recognize that you have a weakness, accept that it's a weakness, and work hard to 'substitute' other pleasures. Moving forward, let's remember that Substitution Therapy is a 'forced distraction', like a horse with blinders on. Your ultimate test of strength comes in facing your temptations head on and walking away unharmed. If you were tired, hungry, and stressed, could you resist the temptation of a tasty restaurant buffet? When situations like this happen, and they always will, you will find that just a small increase in your level of impulse control will help. Outside the arena of confrontational situations like the one I just mentioned, Substitution Therapy must become your salvation. My advice here is to become a student of human behavior so you can discover your own internal motivators and your own passions, so you, too, can distract yourself for most of your waking hours.

I have made a fairly bold statement with the title of this book, 'The Untold Secrets of Permanent Weight Loss'. It would appear as that I am no different than any other financial predator in search of all the desperate dieters of the world. Almost. Here's where everything should fall into place for you. You must find **your** distractions and follow through with your own plan if you want permanent weight loss. If you think reading a book will be the answer, then you are lazy and missing a valuable point. Your issues, your faulty thinking, your denial - they all must be addressed, and addressed by you for changes to be permanent. It is only when you have successfully de-programmed yourself that any kind of dietary change will become a daily habit instead of a daily struggle. Are we clear on this?

## Meditation and Visualization

To most of us, the power of the human mind is inconceivable. We rarely test our strength and potential to achieve great things in our lives. Why? Because if you have never tapped into your strength on a grand scale, you can never know of it's existence. Your mind is so strong that it can be the source of your liberation, or your destruction, yet most of us tend to deny its potential.

You can connect to your own dormant 'inner strength' through the common process of meditation. Spend thirty minutes each day in reflection, where there is a conscious effort to eliminate negative thoughts and emotions, and bridge the connection to your true 'soul', where a feeling of well being will dominate. It may seem fruitless and 'a little too eastern', but learning to meditate, or at least void out your environment and focus on absolutely nothing, is a valid mental exercise. If you perform this and accomplish this, even on a minor level, the emotions of contentment, pleasure, and wonder will bring your energy and ability to focus to a place you never thought possible. I can tell you with the utmost confidence that everyone who is overweight has some form of 'self image' problem with almost no energy and few positive convictions. Meditation is a true remedy for faulty thinking and a vital catalyst for your goal of permanent weight loss. Learn it as though your happiness and quality of life depend on it, because they do.

Let's look at 'visualization' and how it can help you stay the course. Visualization is your mind's ability to take you to the end of your journey, to a place where the end result has already occurred. It is truly a potent and positive form of connecting with the true strength of your mind. Athletes visualize the end result of their activities, actors their performances, and successful business people visualize their financial achievements. You can use it to 'see' into your own future management of your weight. **Visualization is important because, before you can accomplish the 'physical' part of your plan, you have to 'lock in' your mind's focus on something that is real and tangible**. It could be a photograph of a physique that you wish to emulate hanging on your wall, a pair of blue jeans in your closet, or any other visual reminder of the path you chose to take. Visualization guides your mind's strength in an almost subconscious way. Your thoughts and actions are guided by visualization, so learn to tap into your own strength, where your dieting and exercise efforts will seem alot less challenging than ever before. Strengthen your mind and everything else you want to accomplish with your life will fall into place. I'll take a book 'How to Visualize' or 'Meditation Exercises' over any diet book, because I can get a grocery list anywhere.

It is our collective mental weakness as a culture that makes us vulnerable to destructive outside forces. The stronger your convictions are, the less you can be influenced by what 'they' tell you will work. The concept of weight loss with little or no responsibility or effort on your part is being pushed hard in today's marketplace. Dependency on others (or drugs) is critical to financial success for all the companies that try to sell you on the idea that we, as a people, cannot take care of ourselves, and that, when left on our own, we will self-destruct. You should now have a clear understanding of how faulty your thinking has been and how important it is to become independent and mentally tough through meditation and visualization. Books on the practice of meditation and visualization can be found in almost any bookstore. The question here becomes one of resistance. Are you willing to take the more challenging path of hard work, success, and commitment to yourself, or continue on the easy path of laziness and quick-fix solutions that fail? Now, let's take a look at the bright side of the task of strengthening your resolve.

## The Joy of Discipline

Let me provide you with a snapshot of my journey and one of the discoveries I made along the way. My original attitude was no different than yours would be, taking to task a new challenge where I had a concept in mind to become leaner, healthier, and more disciplined. I made a list of everything I experienced emotionally that was negative, and there was a lot of it. All these things that contributed to my misery - frustration, resentment, envy, blaming others for my own shortcomings, and a general feeling of dissatisfaction, all became lost baggage for me and contentment and joy seemed to flow internally for no reason. Ah, but there was a reason. The 'practice' of discipline alone - controlling only what was in my domain to control, becoming a free and independent thinker, and, for the most part, putting my ego in the back seat, opened up a door I never expected. I became a happy person. Being in control became so intensely satisfying that I started to enjoy every minute of every day, and in almost a childlike fashion, I gained a new energy and appreciation for life. If you make a conscious attempt to conquer your own faulty reasoning, the results will be the same for you. **The by-product of your newfound discipline will be a strong sense of well- being and contentment.** This end result can and will occur in your life too, but you have to embrace it without hesitation and stay on course. It is truly a bold claim on my part, but I challenge you to work on your own psychological challenges and discover anything different.

Now, in addition to a leaner, healthier you, there is more reason than ever for you to escape from your distorted outlook on what discipline can produce in your own life. Most of us, when we set a goal, enjoy the achievement or 'end result' of our goal, but not the journey that took us there. Understand that your enjoyment will come from both your journey and the arrival at your destination.

### Five Steps of Empowerment

If you are serious and willing to honestly evaluate yourself, there is a reward offered for your effort. To get to this 'place' in your mind, you have no choice but to eliminate any way of retreating from these challenges.

All pathways to failure have to be 'blocked off'. How do you do this? By simply burning every bridge of retreat from your current flawed mode of thinking. You must force yourself into having no alternative but to move forward to a favored outcome or self-destruct with what you know is irrational thinking and imaging. Let's look at how you can develop your own internal strength.

**Step 1. Question Everything.** Everything you know or think you know about healthy eating habits, what is good or bad, what you were told in the past, and what you see and hear now, must be suspect. You must develop a 'resistance to acceptance' through the process of being independent with your thinking. Remember, once you are under the influence of others (a slave), your impulses become much harder to control. Understand that other people, as well as your environment, may influence you, but they do not control you. Eliminate the faulty reasoning that allows you to think that other people and your environment are to blame. They are not. If you fall into the trap of blindly following the majority, where it is believed that dieting is easy and impatience is acknowledged and rewarded, your challenge will overwhelm you and you will quit in frustration. Start believing in yourself. Again, lose your motivation to become a 'conformist' in a collectively overweight society.

**Step 2. Evaluate and Accept Yourself.** Develop your ability to see flaws in your thinking and reach an honest level of understanding about yourself. It is critical that you have the ability so 'see' yourself rationalizing poor habits and behavior regarding nutrition and exercise. Make a list of other pleasures or passions in your life so they can be magnified and dominate your need to eat for the wrong reasons. Acceptance of the role you play in determining your own future is also critical. If you can't progress beyond the passive stance of denial about what you can control, your self-assessment will have no foundation and you will fail.

**Step 3. Eliminate Your Resistance.** Specifically, your resistance to change. You must conquer the mental anguish (fear) that comes with forced change. Although your change will be positive, you and I both fear it. It's a journey into the unknown, so resistance is our natural response. Conquering these irrational fears is accomplished through mental exercises that include some form of meditation and visualization. Change is good. Once you understand how to 'catch yourself' from resisting and learn how to consistently identify it, doors will open for you and 'free will' won't be such a destructive force. Understand that your 'inner voice' can be a corrupting influence, and allows you to rationalize and fabricate excuses. You must be able to break through this barrier. Chapter Seven of this book covers the pain involved in change and what you must do to overcome it.

**Step 4. Educate Yourself.** Not much need for explanation here. Ignorance about nutrition and exercise only serves to provide you with an 'out', so to speak. With knowledge comes enlightenment and power, so becoming pro-active with your quest for knowledge is vital to your success. How much do you know about human behavior? What about your own behavior? Add these answers to your new list of things to learn. It is absolutely critical that you have some basic understanding of human nature. You can't manage the motivators behind your own impulses until you become a student again. The 'ignorance bridge' of retreat has to be burned if you are to move forward.

**Step 5. Set a 'Flawed' Pathway to a Long Term Goal.** Manage yourself as the irrational human that you are. Constant internal conflict will eventually sabotage any long- term effort. Giving yourself a margin for error keeps the frustration and feelings of self-disgust from totally breaking you down. It is also important, too, that when you allow yourself to go off track, you come to a peaceful resolution about the guilt you may feel. Visualization should also play a key role in reaching your goals. Remember what I told you about tangible results. Make it something you can see and create imagery in process of your effort. Bring a 'balanced' approach to your quest to shed those extra pounds permanently. Understand too, that impatience and unrealistic expectations (what the 'experts' are telling you) undermine your focus.

## The Perfect Diet Defined

Up to this point, your understanding of what pre-determines your success should be obvious. If there is so much deception in the industry, then how will you and I know how to filter out all this bad information? After all, there is a diet plan that is superior to all others. In my case, I spent the last twenty years experimenting, changing, buying into false claims, and finally reaching the conclusion, as you will too, that groceries are secondary to your primary plan to treat yourself as a mortal human being with limited powers. What is the best diet for you? It's the diet that becomes habit by day one thousand, and it's the diet that 'regulates' your cheating and keeps you in a balanced state. It's an evolved way of thinking, where, in your mind, eating becomes a science instead of a form of 'sensory gratification'. Most of the time, anyway. To be honest here, let's agree that the perfect diet has very little to do with food. **It's a building process of self-control over time that evolves from conscious to sub-conscious behavior through repetition**. **Understand?** This is your one and only roadmap to success. If you must, highlight this paragraph or copy it and post it on your refrigerator. It's that critical. A perfect analogy for this conscious to subconscious model would be the way you drive your car now. In the beginning, you had to focus on all the details and your stress levels were much higher. You consciously thought of braking, accelerating, turning, merging, etc. How do you drive your car now? That's right. It's all subconscious habit. Auto-pilot, you might say. If you are willing to drive these new diet principles into your thinking, they too will become subconscious action as time progresses. Again, this takes effort on your part, and the pay-off is not immediate. If you are lazy and want a grocery list, refer to the thousands of diet books that offer terrific nutritional advice. If you want results, start right now, eliminate, for example, trash carbohydrates(processed sugars and starches) from your diet for only three days. If you catch any flack from friends, family, or co-workers, laugh it off, and refer back to the self-empowerment principles. If you started today, worked up a list of reasons why your eating habits are so poor, identified the sources of your excesses, and began a simple five day on, two day off routine, by year two all of this struggle for inner dominance will become subconscious habit, and that, my friend, is the perfect diet.

## Crunch Time

By now I should have you thinking about your past efforts and what may have caused them to fail or yield results that you felt were unacceptable. All these engrained beliefs, attitudes, and behavior patterns from your past have to be under scrutiny. Remember that short- term efforts are easy and do nothing for you in relation to managing the rest of your life. Over time, your long -term effort will become less of a struggle and your thinking will evolve into habit, where internal conflict is almost completely eliminated. If you are truly serious about changing your life, and I suspect you are, write down your own long- term goal. I suggest a 'One Year' plan. It may only take six months to achieve the physical results you want, but your effort to 'de-program' yourself will take all the time and discipline you are willing to invest.

## Chapter 4

### Your Realistic Plan

The first order of business you need to address here is that common American cultural belief that you can change 'instantly'. Read my lips. It ain't happening. There is no quick fix or 'ice cream and pizza' diet plan. From this point forward, the words 'fast' and 'quick' should not exist in your vocabulary of weight loss terms. Stop buying into the hype. There is only you and your ability be patient, and understand that climbing a mountain is not a sprint. I know you become frustrated when results come too slow, but that's just the way it is. Again, you have to stop listening to what 'they' tell you regarding expectations. Now that you are hopefully living in the real world, look back on the last ten years, and see the subtle changes in your diet and exercise habits and how they have contributed to your status today. My point here is that you may have put on twenty pounds (numbers are irrelevant) over ten years. Taking those twenty pounds off in ten days is a pipe dream! Even ten weeks is a challenge. You spent the last 520 weeks packing it on, so be realistic. Most doctors recommend a pace of about one to two pounds per week for anyone that is not obese. If that's not fast enough for you, then you have patience issues, my friend. Most diets start out with more weight loss in the first month, then a tapering off as you approach your ideal weight. Use common sense here. If you are severely overweight and plan to take a drastic approach to weight loss, I highly recommend doing it under a doctor's supervision.

**The right pace.** The human body is fascinating in its own attempt to survive without your influence. As you lose weight, dropping from, for example, 20 percent body fat down to 10 percent, your body does make it more difficult to lose additional weight due to its ability to stabilize. It's a survival mechanism we all have. This translates to a rate of loss that will decrease over time. Remember this and factor it into your own plan. It's natural for your body to stabilize as you approach your ideal weight. Again, your thinking is flawed if, on the ninth week of diet, you lose only half a pound, and you consider this failure because you have a history of losing

61

two pounds per week. You must understand your own history of weight gain. Slow, gradual weight gained over the course of ten years presents a much greater challenge than the pounds you put on over the holidays. If it takes a year for you to reach your goal, then so be it. Don't fall prey to the promise of 'instant' success. "They", meaning, the media, the Diet Plan Companies, Magazines, Books, and Videos, have a reputation for setting you and I up for failure. When you set a goal or develop a plan that turns out to be unrealistic, your self-confidence and drive take it right on the chin. One failed attempt after another can become habit, and every attempt you make in the future will fail because you expect failure as an end result. Is this a familiar scenario? Remember what I said about patience. Put yourself in a position to reach your goal. Live with the happy people in the village of reality.

**Plan for imperfection.** None of us can claim to be superhuman. Allow for some decadent meals and snacks on occasion. It may actually work in your favor to take one day per week and give in to what you have been craving for days. Your direction is more important than your speed here. So what if you only lost one pound last week. You **are** losing weight, so beating yourself up over it is self-defeating. Let's not make dieting any more stressful than it has to be. A few restaurant meals every now and then can be very enjoyable. You should plan to go off the track. In a typical week, you may want to take one or two days and allow yourself to satisfy some cravings. Try four days on, and one day off. If you need to increase it to five days on, one day off, then do it, but do it with conviction. These 'valves' are necessary in dealing with your human side, so you need to be flexible and develop an attitude of eating for pleasure on occasion without the side order of guilt. By forgiving yourself, you can now truly enjoy those dinners at your favorite local restaurant or any other indulgence of culinary kind.

**Avoiding negative influences.** The downside to our nature relative to interaction with others is that we often want people to fail. It's not to be harmful, but if you fail with your attempts to reach your goal, you now become one of us. One of the majority. You are now a member of the society of excess. Welcome, friend, we so love your contribution to our collective ignorance. Ah, a place to call home. Not quite. After all, haven't most of the people you know failed with their own attempts to lose weight permanently? We all want to identify with each other, and validating your own identity with 'most of society' makes us feel normal, and human. That is why most of us tend to view overly ambitious, hard-working, or highly self disciplined people with a suspicious eye. We have trouble with the identification process, so, in turn, our attitude is tainted with negativity, and we fail to empathize with people who are not 'mainstream' in their behavior like the rest of us. Even well wishing family and friends will subconsciously, or in some cases, openly attempt to sabotage your efforts. Be aware that not everyone will embrace your new disciplined lifestyle. It can be tough to go it alone, but you must. Sure, it's great if someone joins you in your challenge, but to depend on that or look for constant support is inviting failure.

In addition to people pressure comes cultural and social pressure. Commercials, billboards, magazines, even big neon signs on the highway invite you to be part of the new American society of excess. The good news is that there is a fork in the road, and you have the internal power to follow the road less traveled, where strength and discipline will be rewarded. You should never feel pressure to fit in. Think and be your own person. Stop playing the role of the conformist. As a whole, our culture, the way it exists now, is not worth emulating.

**Control and minimize stress.** Stress truly is a negative influence on all of us. Americans are often overstressed. Our lifestyle is fast-paced, and our culture is competitive by nature. The only way to minimize stress is to understand it. Remember what I said about control. Be in control of what you can, but forget about what you can't. When you think about stress from a psychological standpoint, most stress is not real. What I mean is that most of your stress is self-imposed. It's what I call phantom stress. Real stress is rare. A twister headed towards your house or someone intent on doing bodily harm to you is real stress(or, in this case, danger). The rest is all in your head.

Even the strongest and most disciplined of us will feel stresses that are unavoidable. The loss of a loved one or being fired from a job tend to induce high amounts of stress. These are not ideal situations for you to think about focusing on your diet. When stress is high, you should concentrate on eliminating it and you may forget about your diet temporarily. There should be no guilt or shame associated with any period of high stress in your life. Stay balanced. Don't try to do the impossible. Do, however, try to seek out activities, situations, or people that have a calming effect on your mental state. By the way, exercising will yield fantastic results in the lowering of stress levels. Make a checklist of things that relax you and intentionally follow through as though your mental well being is a project in itself.

**Re-direct your passions.** This is the part of our collective quest that comes back to bite most of us right in the ass. As I explained earlier, your focus on pleasing yourself with tasty meals and treats has to be diverted. Don't expect me to hold your hand and walk you through this part. The ball is in your court here. You know what you are passionate about, and you must intensify one or many of your other desires, or you will fail. You will fail because will power on its own will eventually break down if a void still exists. Your support group is not going to be a relative, a friend, or a co-worker. It's going to be your exploration into other things that motivate and excite you. The void must be filled.

**The critical element of balance.** No one person is perfectly in sync with the universe, but many of us are more 'balanced' in our approach to life and its challenges, and that's a good thing. By 'balanced', I mean having things in perspective. Being somewhat organized. Being in control and recognizing the signs of imbalance. Many of us have obsessive tendencies with our attitudes towards eating. **When you ignore your own health to gratify an obsessive desire to eat, that's a major imbalance!** You must be critical of yourself and have the ability to 'catch' yourself when you fall into obsessive behavior. Failing to control our desires and urges leads to a multitude of behavioral problems and severely irrational thinking. Balance has to be present everywhere. A balanced diet, a balanced daily schedule of work and play, a balanced family life. Balanced people understand the need for proper nutrition and exercise. They don't beat themselves up or give up their challenge over one day's indulgence. They understand and accept their human side. Identify with the balanced people around you. Learn to observe their behavior, their actions, their speech, and make an attempt to become one of these people. These people make good role models, but the initiative to educate yourself and develop new habits must be accomplished by you alone. After all, if your life is balanced, it is a result of your own intentions and efforts, and if you can get to this place emotionally, chances are you have migrated from slave to master.

## Goal Setting

Now you must put your discipline to the test. Anytime change is going to occur, and that change requires a dose of self -control, some type of criteria of measurement has to be established. Setting your own personal goals for changing your eating habits requires self-analysis, but I can definitely help you with the mechanics. Let's look at how to go about setting goals you can achieve.

**Set a long- term goal and break it down into segments of short term goals.** There is a lot of credence to the use of 'baby steps'. Remember, what you are trying to accomplish is an attempt to reverse years of poor habits and attitudes, so take it slow and methodically. To be impatient here is to be foolish. No stomach stapling or prescriptions for stimulants are necessary. Start out with a flexible weekly goal, and build in a safety valve or two. If you are only eating two meals a day now, then increase to three in the beginning. Going back to the issue of pace, your own healthy, manageable rate of weight loss will probably fall between one to two pounds per week. Set a weekly goal that is conservative for you. A goal of one to two pounds per week sounds attainable and not overwhelming for your level if you are, in fact, overweight. Losing twenty five pounds in three months appears to be a difficult challenge until you break it down to weekly objectives. You are in unfamiliar territory, so knowing how your body will respond can be unpredictable. If you lose only one pound in a week where your goal was two, you are still moving in the right direction. Losing four pounds in one week may be the feedback you need to perhaps spend one or two days a week being a little less disciplined and treating yourself a few times. Baby steps.

**Flexibility.** Okay, so you are on the righteous path of weight loss and content with your weekly results.

Then tragedy strikes. A week of hardcore dieting yields almost no results. You are a complete failure. You will die homeless and broke, and no one will love you. This response is a little on the unbalanced side, but it proves my point. Standing on the scale four times a day, measuring foods with laboratory beakers, and 'obsessing' is self- destructive. Set a target goal, aim for the bulls eye, but if you miss, you miss. Be content to be on the target. Remember what I told you about your own body's reaction to dieting. As your level of body fat decreases, so does the pace of weight loss. As weeks or months go by, it does get tougher, so flexibility in dealing with results is critical. You must adjust on the fly. If you must re-set your weekly goal to a half a pound, then a half a pound it is. Stay the course. Be patient. You may want to allow for a week-long break if you're going on vacation and planning to eat out most of that week. Avoid the temptation to look outside for the new and different. There is no super-high-energy-eat-all-you-want-lose-ten-pounds-a-week-diet plan. Let's move on.

## Chapter 5

## The G.O.Y.A. Principles of Exercise

Over the course of the last, say, fifty years, our culture has lost its way on the path to health and fitness. If 25 million people say they don't have the time to exercise, then it must be true. Right? Wrong. I call it a collective faulty rationale that has crept into the psyche of our society and spread like a cancer. The President of the United States, as busy as he is, finds time to exercise. Here is another fact about our nature as humans. **We always find time to do the things we really want to do.** This includes you, too, my friend. 'I've been too busy' is a conditioned response now, just as saying 'Hi, how are you doing?' If your life is filled with all the typical pursuits of money, education, love, social status, family obligations, the accumulation of power, etc., with no room for exercise, then you need to re-evaluate your values. I say this with complete confidence because without quality of life, the other trappings become meaningless. But it's your defective programming at the core of your resistance. May I be so bold to say that you, as a reader of this book, are a liar. A big liar. We are all liars. Everyone will rationalize their decision making and their behavior from time to time. We lie to ourselves. Some more than others.

Again, I will stress that to look outside yourself for answers or enlightenment is dangerous and will only yield negative results. The drill instructor you wish would instill discipline in you, live with you, maybe even force you to exercise three to four times a week, is a fabrication. It's our nature to shift blame from ourselves or to look outside for answers. **Your excuse for being inactive is usually anything but the truth**. That's where the GOYA principles come into play. What does GOYA stand for? It stands for **"Get Off Your Ass"**. If you were expecting maybe a miracle phrase that would force you into a moment of enlightenment, you were wrong. Of course, this phrase has been around for years. I must credit Tom Hopkins, whose book on Selling first introduced this GOYA principle. It is the most valid and simple one I know. Do not let your own ignorance stop you, either. That's a cop out, too. Exercise comes in all forms. Take some initiative and learn a few things about resistance training, aerobics, yoga, swimming, or any other form of exercise. Again, get off your ass. 'I hate exercise' is a statement made by a fool and ignorance is no excuse either. 'I don't have the time' is a lie many of us tell ourselves over and over again to rationalize lack of motivation or even to cover up irrational fears. What this statement really means is ' I refuse to sacrifice the time'. Remember, everyone, including you, can find the time. I know that, internally, you may feel justified with your work, family, and social obligations, but keep in mind the element of balance and your pre-disposed desire to fit in with society. Development of your independent 'self' is critical here. You may need to force the issue with segmenting your time or even taking time for yourself if that is the case. Understand that to be the best 'you' you can be - healthy, energetic, happy, and at your personal best- there has to be some downtime. Refer back to the Master-Slave analogy and it will help you to understand and prioritize your time. If you are not in the habit of taking this personal time, then block it off on your calendar and do it intentionally, but do it and do it now. A lie repeated a thousand times as the truth is still a lie, so examine your decision making processes that have failed you over the years. The real world waits to welcome you with arms wide open, so work on breaking down this 'resistance' your own mind has fabricated.

Now that you are off your ass (or at least planning to get off your ass), let's go over some simple guidelines regarding exercise. First and foremost, for losing body fat, the best form of activity is a low impact, long- term session that raises your heartbeat and increases your breathing. Walking for twenty or thirty minutes is a very low impact activity that almost anyone can do. Again, if you have been sedentary for quite some time, you should consult a doctor before starting an exercise regimen. Remembering the need for carbohydrates as fuel, think of short, bursting movements, like tennis or baseball, as carbohydrate burning. Constant stopping and going can be slightly effective for weight loss, but long term, sustained movement is the best. If you are in terrible condition now, start out slow. Maybe a ten-minute walk. After a few weeks, increase to fifteen or twenty minutes. Even low impact swimming will be effective if combined with a sensible diet. If you are more than forty pounds overweight, you may have no choice but to start out with low impact walking or swimming. Your ability to set and be realistic with yourself and your goals comes into play here too.

In a perfect world, you, as the perfect human that you are, would exercise virtually every day. Two sessions of low impact and three sessions of resistance training each week (my preference). You will take in carbohydrates and protein before resistance training (weight training), and perform your low impact sessions on an empty stomach for maximum results. Why so much weight training? Because you want to burn more calories while at rest. Going back to the fat cell versus muscle cell analogy, you should now know that, at rest, you will burn far more calories if you were to pack on a pound or two of muscle. If you are a woman, and concerned with looking hard and masculine if you train with weights, don't be. It's not going to happen. Big weights and long sessions are not necessary. Besides, your testosterone levels are naturally too low.

Let's bring balance back into the picture. If exercising is good, than more would be better, right? Wrong. Other than our collective impatience to gain immediate results from exercise, a key de-motivator for many is the issue of over training(too much exercise). If its been a few years since you hit the gym or the running track, you have no other choice but to progress slowly and listen to your own 'biofeedback'. Exercise is a form of stress that your body needs time to recuperate from. Your body's downtime between workouts is more critical than the workout itself. Getting plenty of rest, water, and proper nutrition is essential. Most trainers agree that the positive results of exercise are mostly due to nutrition, proper rest, and a reduction of stress levels that occur **between** workouts. The company that produces the infomercial on the latest and greatest exercise device is not going to tell you this. Why? Because it's too challenging and the results are not immediate. They rely on our collective ignorance by showing a lean, muscular, model (male or female) involved in a demonstration, and many of us fail to see the smoke and mirrors. What's the hidden agenda? Money, of course. Certainly not the truth, and definitely not reality. You don't need machinery to do abdominal crunches or sit-ups. And if you want to achieve the look of the chiseled model in the advertisement, it's your diet that gets you there, with exercise playing the secondary role. Understand that the thinking, planning, purchasing, cooking, and eating of food consume much of your daily life. Three hourly sessions of exercise each week are a secondary focus in the dimension of time. If you want the 'six pack' look, you may need to set a long term goal, because your percentage of body fat has to decrease dramatically. Sorry, but there is just no other way. Keep in mind that a balanced, moderate approach is the best way to start. In the world of fitness, there are two major causes for failure in beginning an exercise program. First, expectations are too high. When you discover that results are slow and steady, and your six-week goal should have been a twelve- week goal, you 'resist' your own psychological need to readjust, so you fail. Second, in your impulsive zest for results, you end up sore and feeling defeated by a poor initial experience simply because you over trained. Believe me, the chronic soreness and potential for injury that result would turn anybody off. Remember what I said earlier about moderation. If you are not exercising now, start slowly, educate yourself, and take a baby step approach.

## Off to the Gym?

Let's go back and look at a characteristic of human behavior. Specifically, your own engrained behavior and beliefs. If you are the typical American, or a product of a similar culture, your childhood is carefree and adults controlled your pace of learning (School) and exercise. In fact, the concept of exercising for health makes no sense to any child. As you get older, however, you learn games and participate in activities that involve exercise. Organized sports may enter the picture. You begin to understand the benefits of exercise. From puberty on, exercise may come in many forms. Team sports and activities in gym class may be relevant to you. The point I make here is that most of us, whether we exercised a lot or very little throughout our youth, adults (coaches, gym teachers, counselors) were typically in control of our schedule and activities. Very few young adults have engrained behavior and the level of self-discipline that is needed to exercise on a regular basis. The influence of your parents, your peers, and your own mental make-up play a role here, too. Remember, too, that role models and other positive influences may or may not exist, and if they do, are you motivated at this moment to observe and emulate these influences? So how is this relevant to you? Well, let's assume you are in the majority, with marginal discipline and desire to be fit and trim. I can also assume with confidence that you have challenges with your own issues of control and priorities regarding exercise. From high school (or college), most of us are on our own and have to grow and learn through trial and error, observation, and a minor commitment to self-education. You know the facts, and you have some form of knowledge of health and fitness, but you fail to act on it in a way that benefits your health. Reversing the trend of your passive youth can be difficult. But it's the most important challenge we all face as we become adults. Remember that your health is the single most important commodity you own. Stop denying that you, in fact, have absolute power over the size and condition of your own body.

Remember what you have read about the two forms of exercise needed in order to maximize your own results. Resistance training, or weight training, in combination with aerobic (fat burning) activity, is by far the most successful way to stay healthy, strong, and in a 'hot-burning engine' mode. The best place to begin is anywhere but your house or garage, however. With marginal discipline, you need to be around others who have the same challenges and goals. To increase your own chance for long-term success, I highly recommend joining a gym, a Y.M.C.A., or just getting involved with others in team sports. What makes you think you will achieve a 'new found discipline' if you make the commitment to purchase a five hundred- dollar super-flex bio-tech fitness machine and put in your garage? Look in the classified section of any newspaper, and you see hundreds of treadmills and other exercise machines for sale. I'm not saying that your membership dues to a health club won't go to waste. I am saying that it's more difficult to fail if your commitment involves being with others who fit your own profile, as well as others who have overcome many bad habits. These dedicated, healthy, and disciplined people are often found in these settings. Remember what I said about role models. You won't find anyone to observe and emulate by secluding yourself. Only a very small percentage of us can make a success out of a 'home gym' or any exercise regimen that you alone initiate independently. The odds are more in your favor if you can leave the distractions of your dwelling. You need to prioritize and 'segment' your time and you will have to make some form of commitment. If you can't make the commitment of money and time that it will take to get 'real' results, then you've just wasted your money on this book, because you, my friend, are still at ground zero. Remember what I said earlier about the lack of role models. There may be only a few, or there may be none. But in a setting where others are committed and exercising, you have a strong foundation for learning through observation and interaction. That is, if you really want to. I can guarantee with certainty that when you grow old and look back on your life, you will never regret the time and money you invested in your own health. Are we clear on this? Let's move on.

**Your Exercise Schedule**

What I recommend, and what you will find to be most rewarding, is the combination of aerobic and resistance training. If you are a beginner, you will want to start out with two or three weekly sessions of twenty to thirty minutes. A Typical schedule for a **beginner** may look something like this:

Monday, Wednesday, Friday - Resistance training
(All muscle groups)
One set of twelve to fifteen repetitions per muscle
group
Thirty minutes of low-impact aerobics (Walk,
Swim, etc.)

The order really does not matter. You may be more comfortable by starting each training session with aerobics. Try to include as many muscle groups as possible with your resistance training. One set of twelve to fifteen repetitions should be enough as a beginner. As you find yourself becoming stronger or more adapted to your routine, you can add an additional set for each muscle group, and increase your aerobic time accordingly.

As you approach the **'Moderate'** level, you will want to break down your training even more, dividing your resistance training into sub-groups and possibly splitting off your aerobic sessions. You may want to include an extra session each week. A more **Moderate** routine would be:

Monday - Lower body training ( Thighs, Calves, Hamstrings), three sets per Muscle group. Abdominal work, three sets of 35 to 50.

Wednesday - Low impact aerobics, 30 to 45 minutes

Friday - Upper body resistance training(Chest, Back, Shoulders, Arms), three sets of Abdominal work, 35 to 50 reps.

Saturday - Low impact aerobics, 30 to 45 minutes

Finally, as you develop into a more specialized program, your body will adapt and recuperate more efficiently. You can begin to increase the number of sets in your resistance training and the number of minutes you spend with low or high impact aerobics. An **'Advanced'** program would break down this way:

Monday - Lower body resistance training ( Thighs, Hamstrings, Calves, Glutes/Butt), six to eight sets per muscle group. Abdominal work, three sets of 50 to 75.

Tuesday - Low impact aerobics, 45 to 60 minutes

Wednesday - Chest and Back resistance training, six to eight sets per muscle group.

Friday - Low or High impact aerobics, 30 to 45 minutes. Abdominal work, three sets.

Saturday - Shoulders and Arms resistance training, six to eight sets per muscle group.

Remember that these schedules are only a **guideline**. You should adapt your own routine based on your level of advancement, and keep in mind that work out days and specific muscle groups can be inter-mixed to fit you personally. My suggestion, before you begin, is to take a hard look at yourself physically. Recognize your weaknesses and strengths. If you are more than forty pounds overweight, you will want to incorporate more aerobics (maybe three times per week) than resistance training. Bear in mind, too, that if you have not been active for a while, you may actually gain a few pounds in the beginning. Let me explain. Exercising a muscle that has been dormant will cause an expansion at the cellular level. More water and nutrients are demanded by your cells, and because your overall mass (Lean muscle tissue) has increased, your weight will increase accordingly. My advice here is to use the mirror as much as the scale to monitor your results. Clothing may fit differently, too. Use all this feedback to gauge your success in addition to the occasional weigh-in. When training with weights, try working on your weak points first during you workout, when your energy level and strength reserves are at their peak.

# Weight Training – The Basics

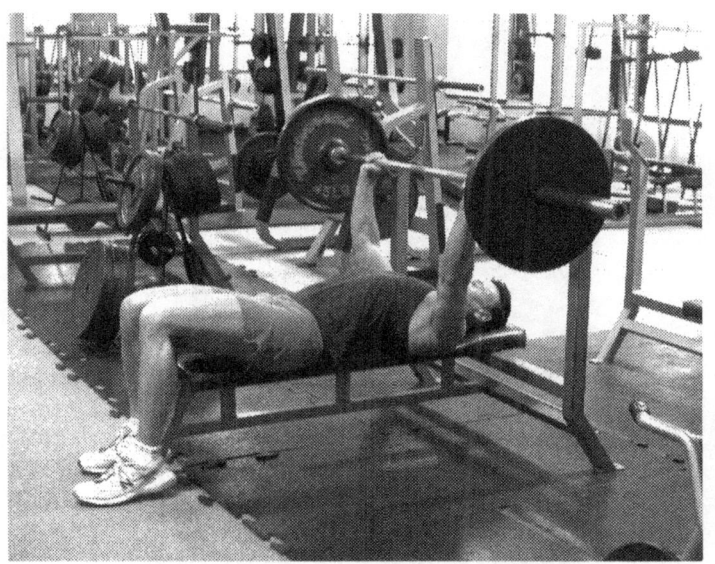

**Chest – Flat Bench Press(Start/Finish)**

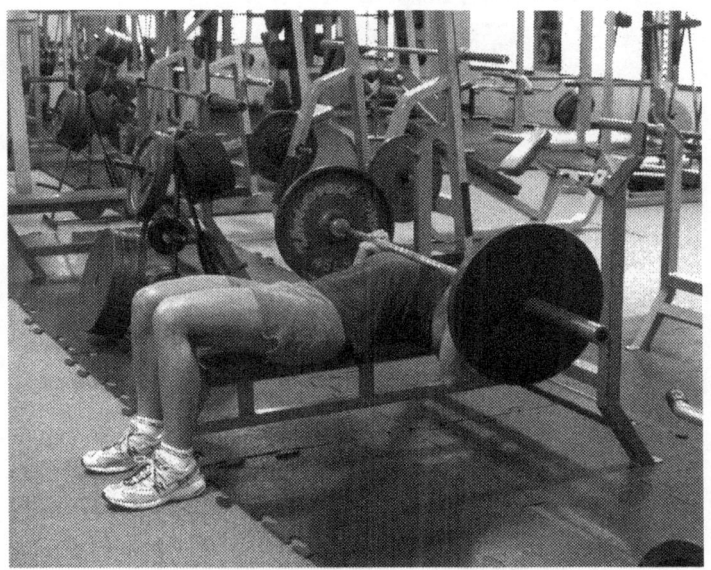

**Chest – Flat Bench Press**

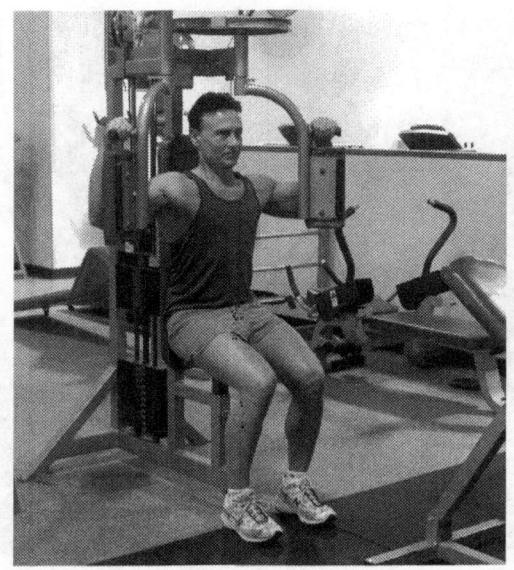

**Chest – Pectoral Machine (Start)**

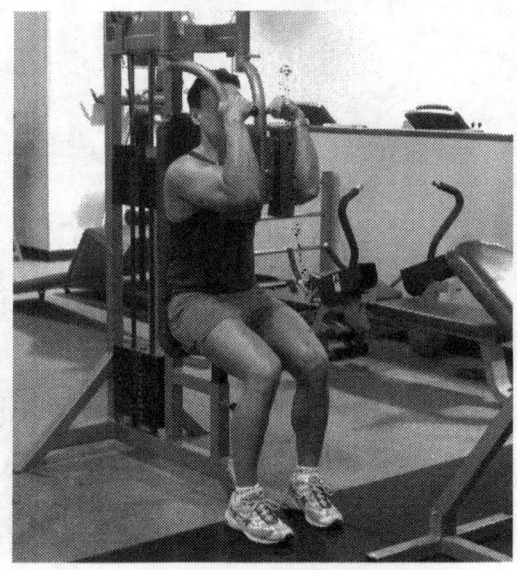

**Chest – Pectoral Machine (Finish)**

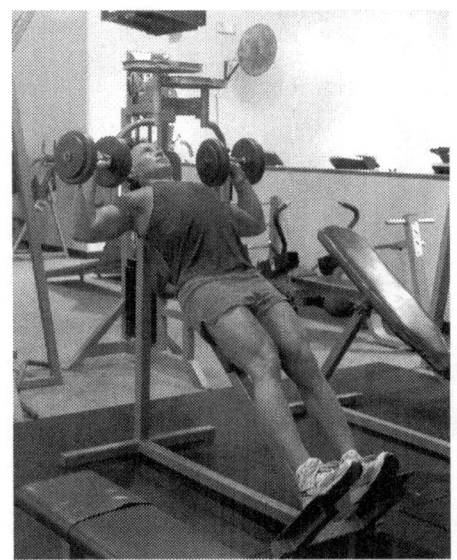

**Chest – Incline Dumbbell Press (Start)**

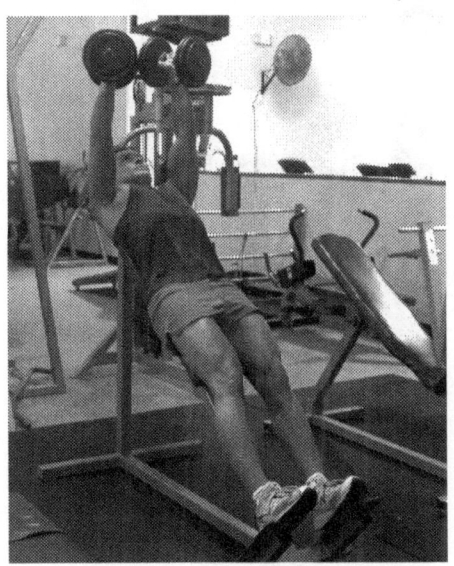

**Chest – Incline Dumbbell Press (Finish)**

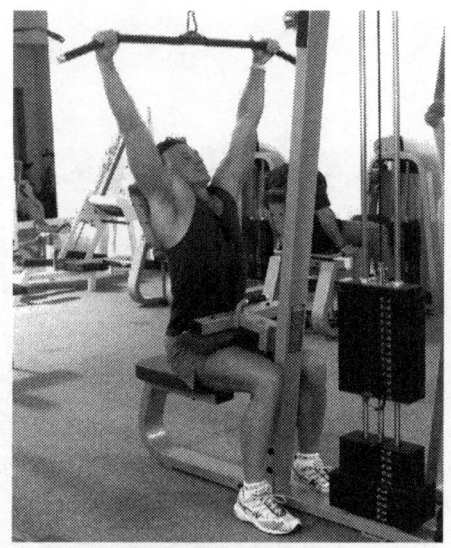

**Back – Lateral Pulldowns (Start)**

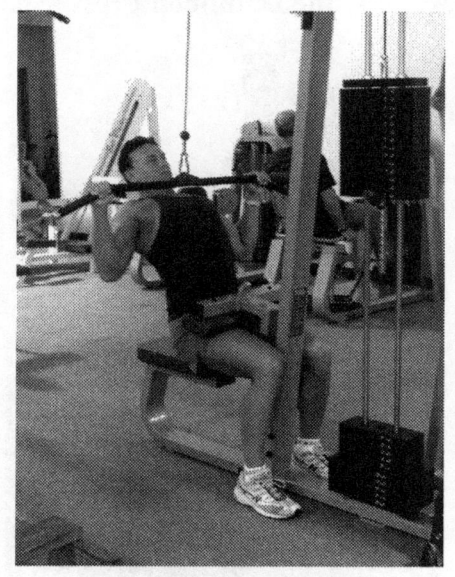

**Back – Lateral Pulldowns (Finish)**

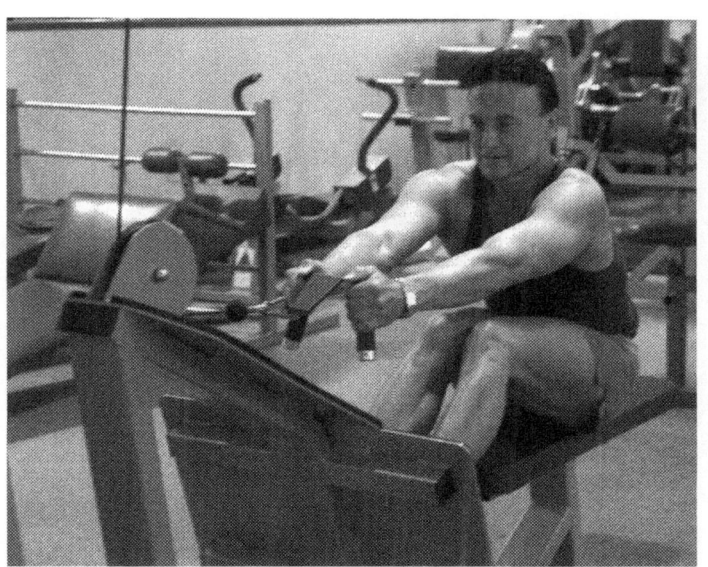

**Back – Cable Rows (Start)**

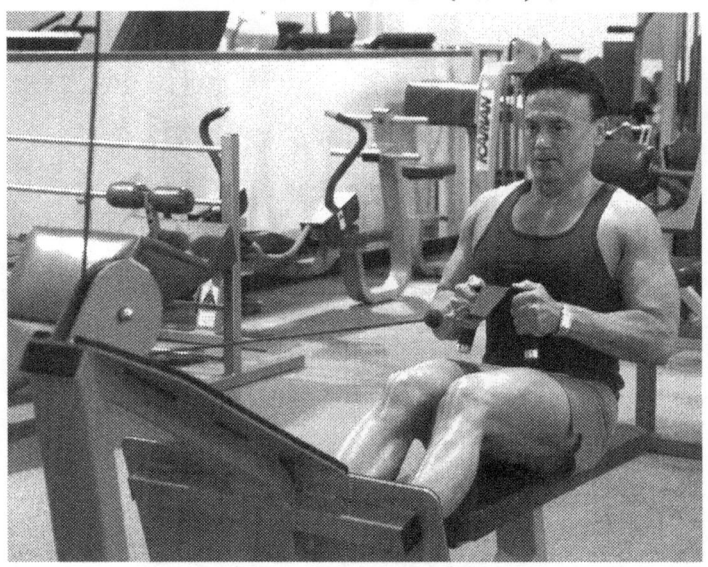

**Back – Cable Rows (Finish)**

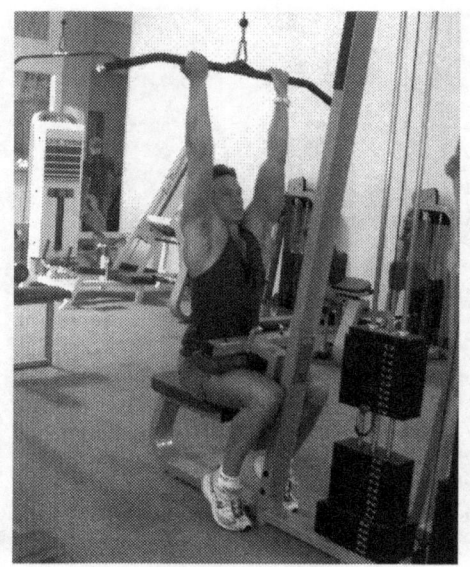

**Back – Close Grip Pulldowns (Start)**

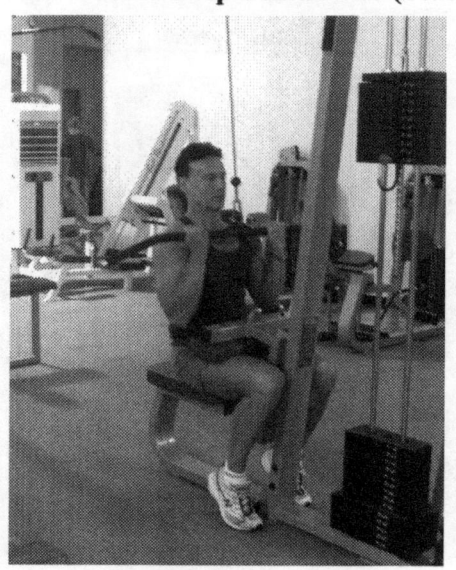

**Back – Close Grip Pulldowns (Finish)**

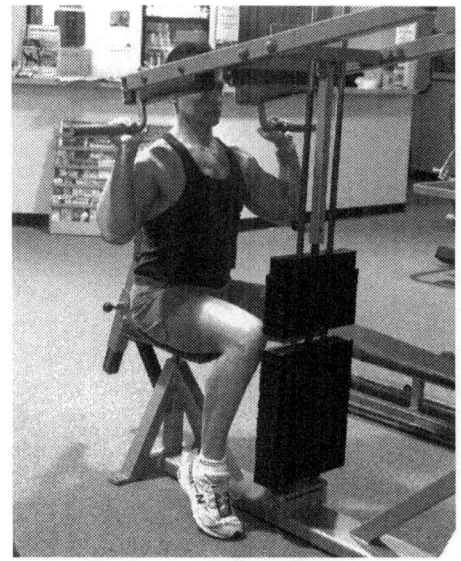

**Shoulders – Military Press (Start)**

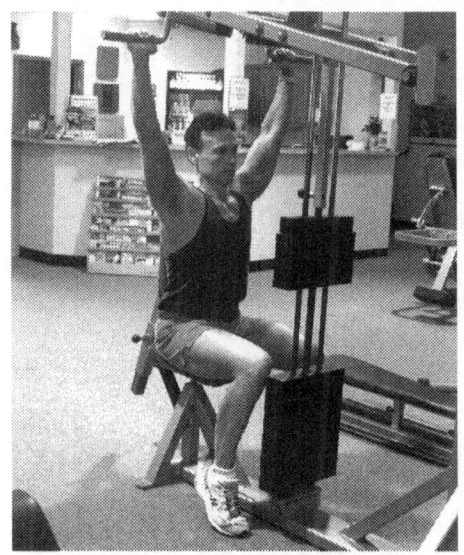

**Shoulders – Military Press (Finish)**

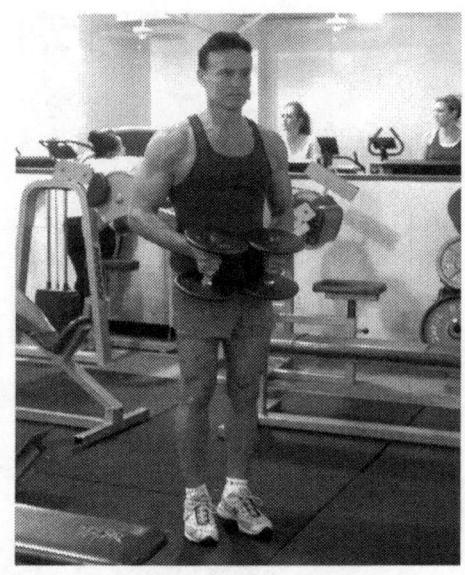

**Shoulders – Lateral Dumbbell Raises (Start)**

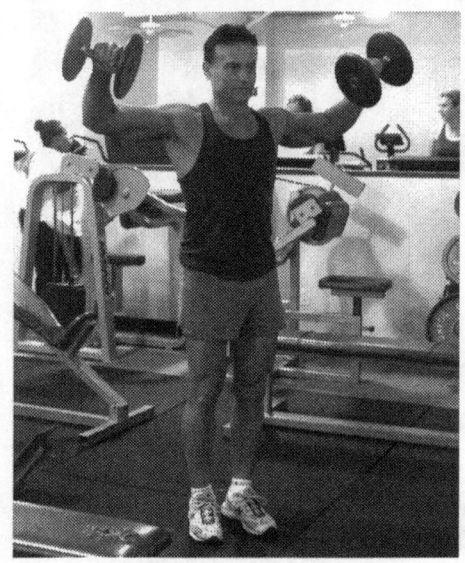

**Shoulders – Lateral Dumbbell Raises (Finish)**

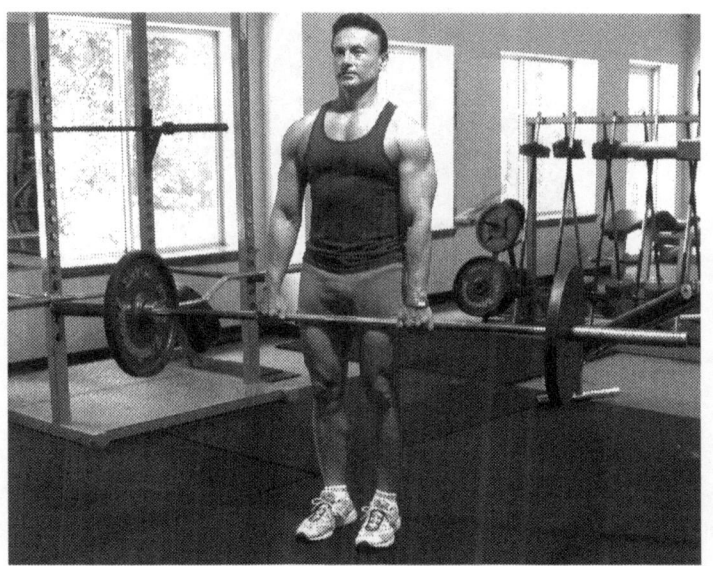

**Shoulders/Traps – Barbell Shrugs (Start)**

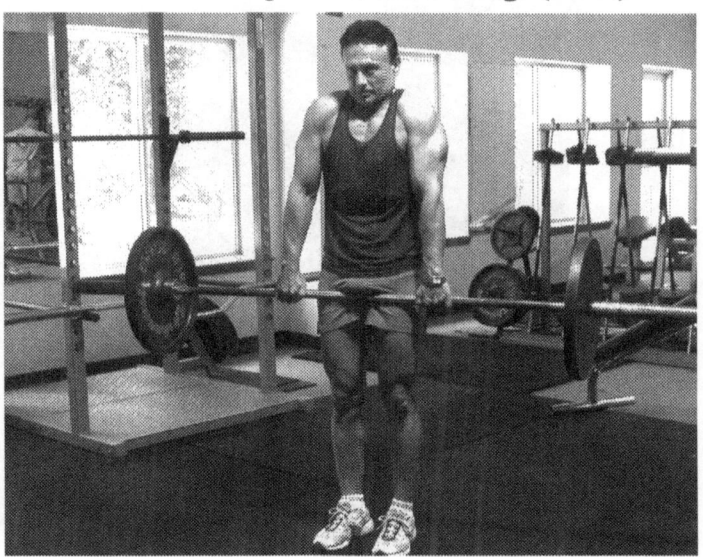

**Shoulders/Traps – Barbell Shrugs (Finish)**

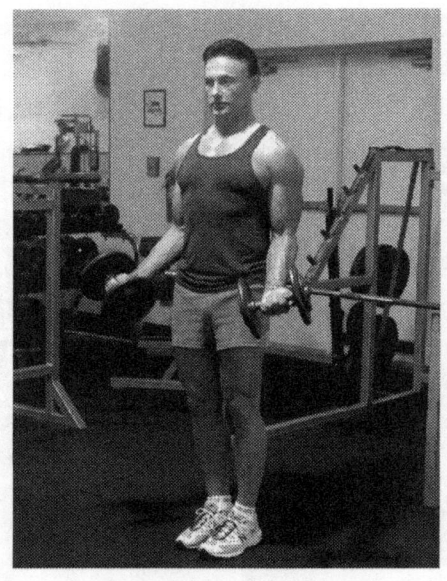

**Biceps/Arms – Standing Dumbbell Curls (Start)**

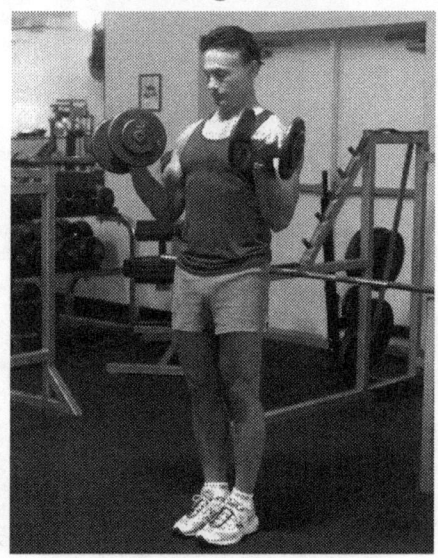

**Biceps/Arms – Standing Dumbbell Curls (Finish)**

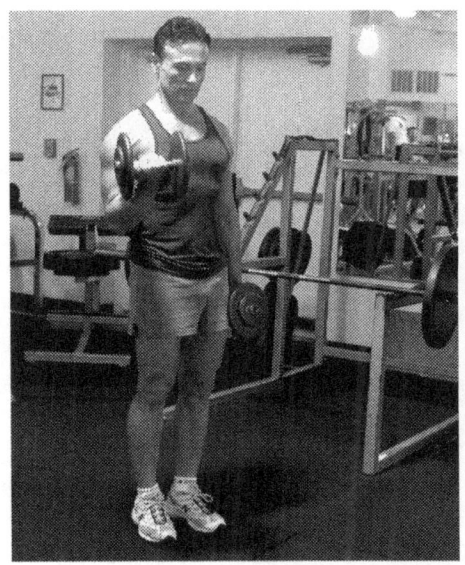

**Biceps/Arms – Alternate Dumbbell Curls (Right)**

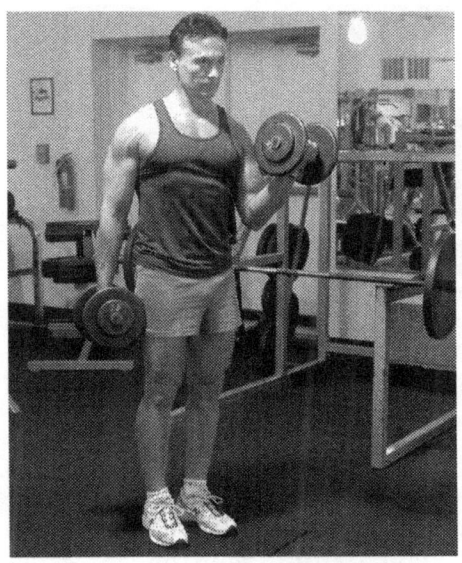

**Biceps/Arms – Alternate Dumbbell Curls (Left)**

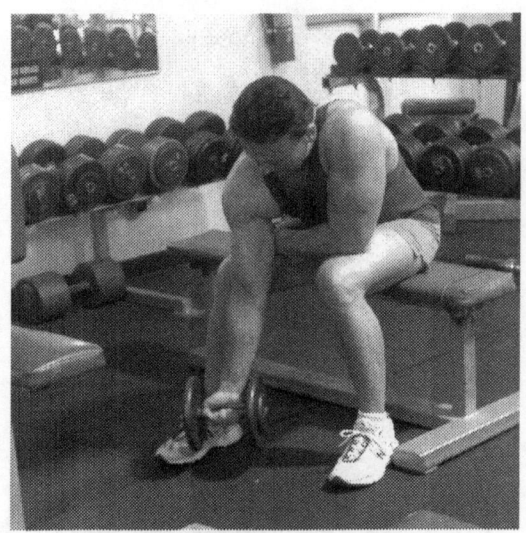

**Biceps/Arms – Dumbbell Concentration Curls
(Start)**

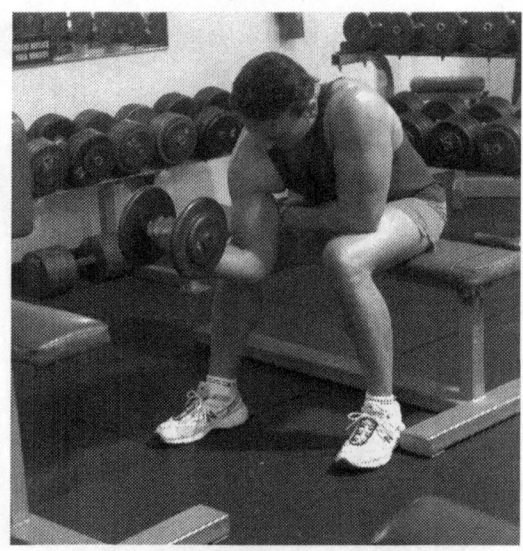

**Biceps/Arms – Dumbbell Concentration Curls
(Finish)**

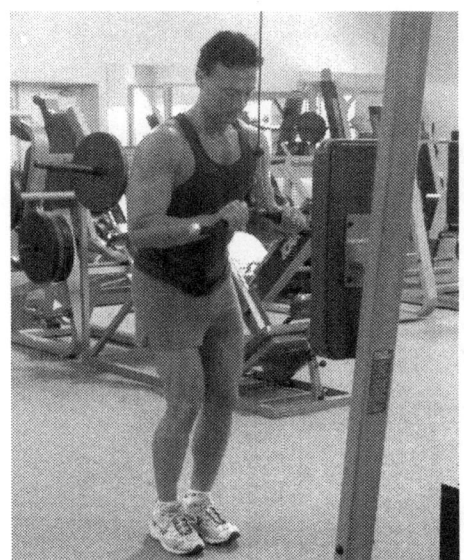

**Triceps/Arms – Cable Pushdowns (Start)**

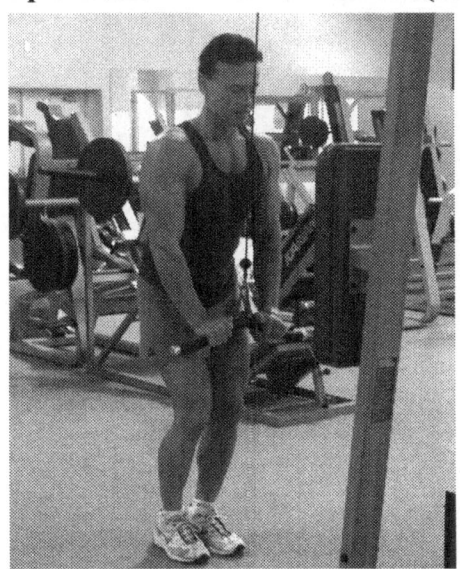

**Triceps/Arms – Cable Pushdowns (Finish)**

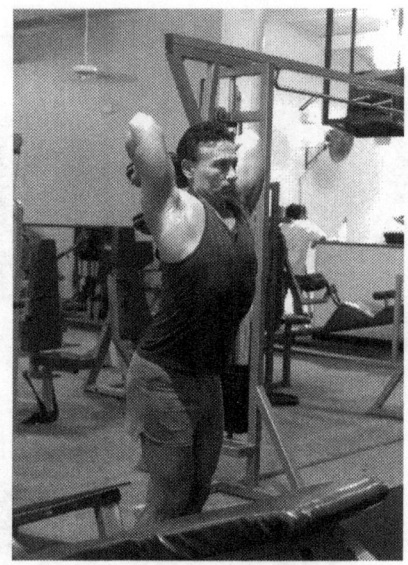

**Triceps/Arms – Dumbbell Raises (Start)**

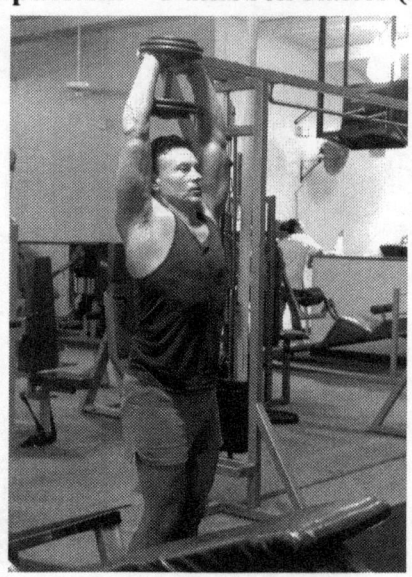

**Triceps/Arms – Dumbbell Raises (Finish)**

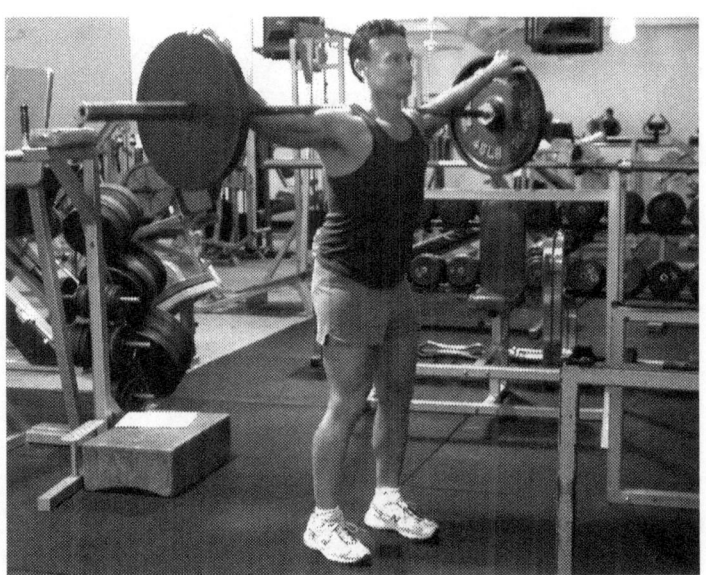

**Legs – Squats (Start/Finish)**

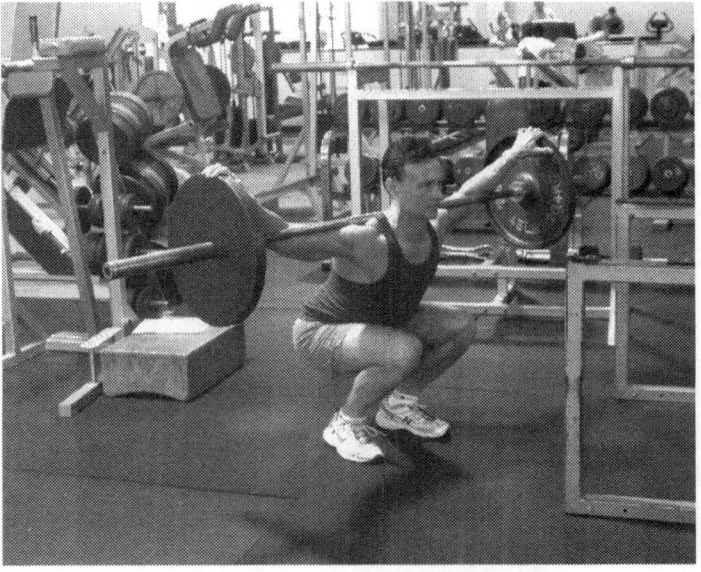

**Legs – Squats (Start/Finish)**

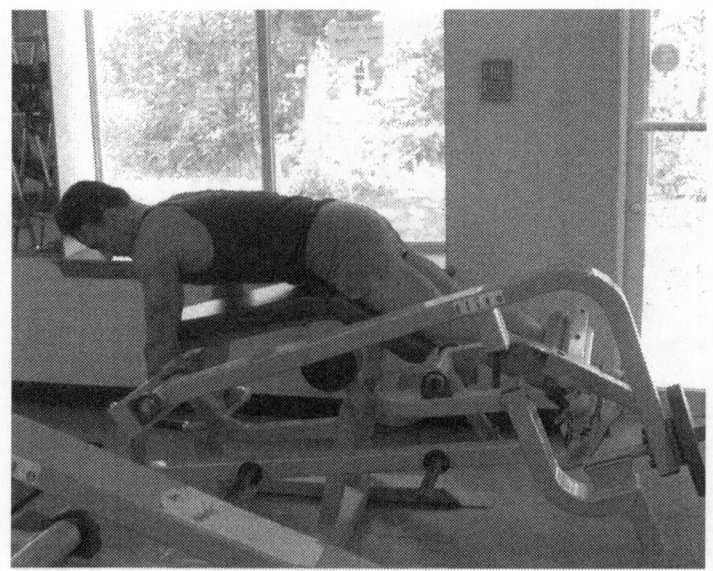

**Hamstrings – Reverse Curls (Start)**

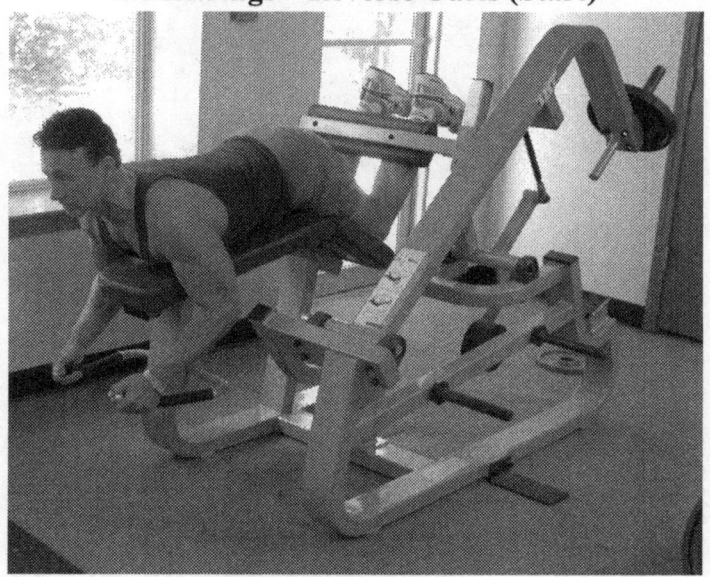

**Hamstrings – Reverse Curls (Finish)**

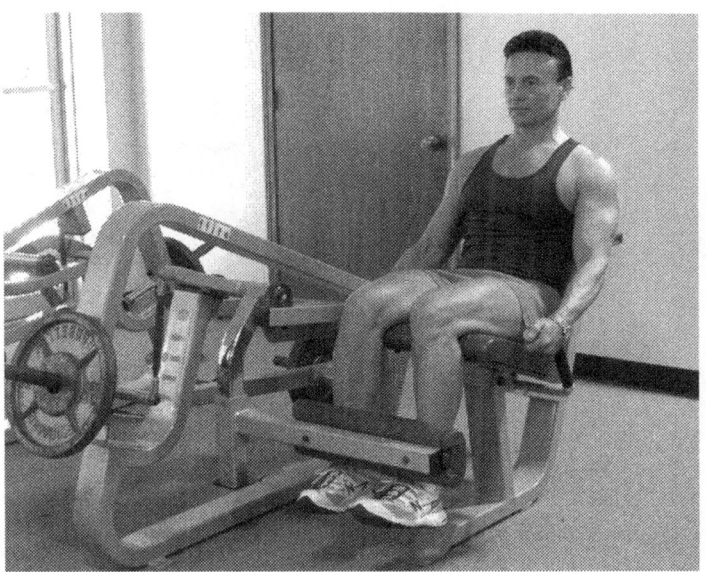

**Thighs – Leg Extension (Start)**

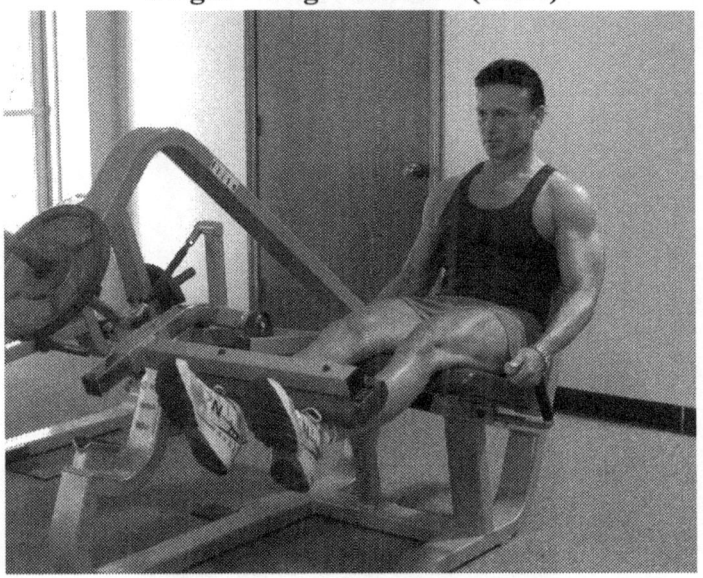

**Thighs – Leg Extension (Finish)**

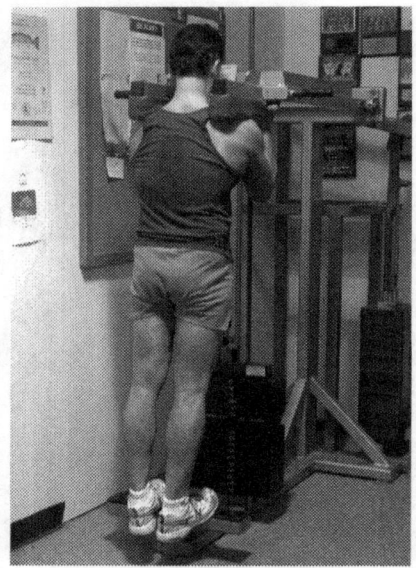

**Calves – Calve Raises (Start)**

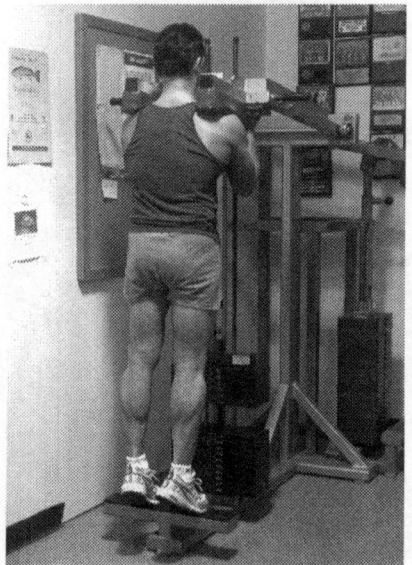

**Calves – Calve Raises (Finish)**

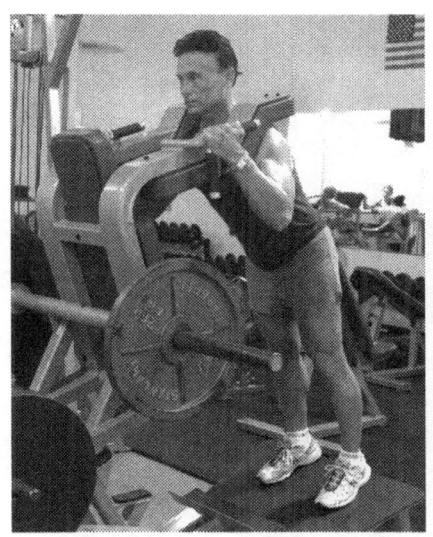

**Legs/ Upper Hamstrings – Reverse Hack Squat (Start/Finish)**

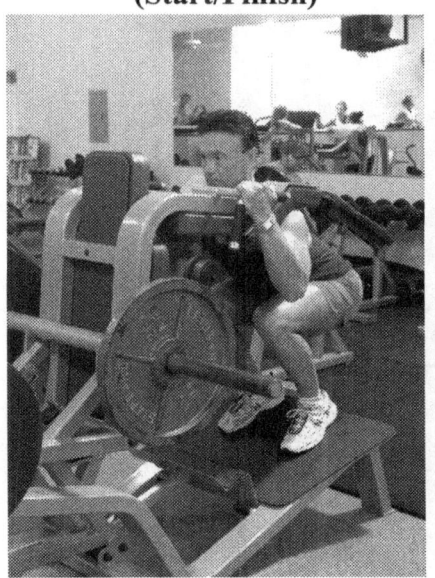

**Legs/Upper Hamstrings – Reverse Hack Squat**

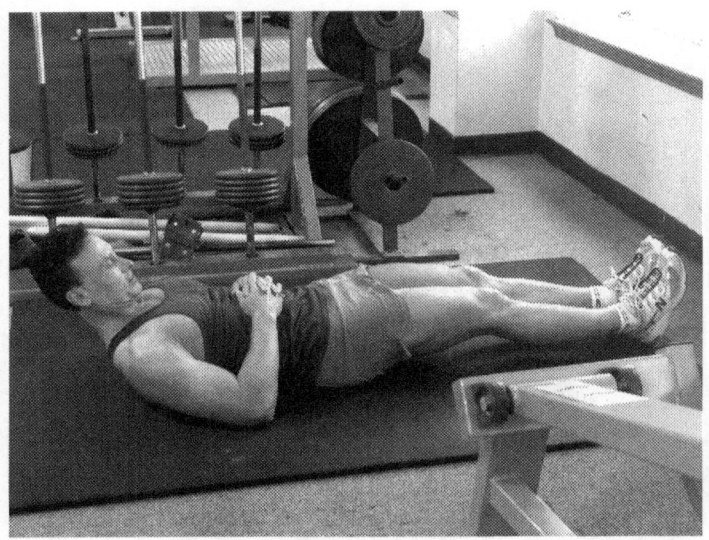

**Abdominals – Crunches (Start)**

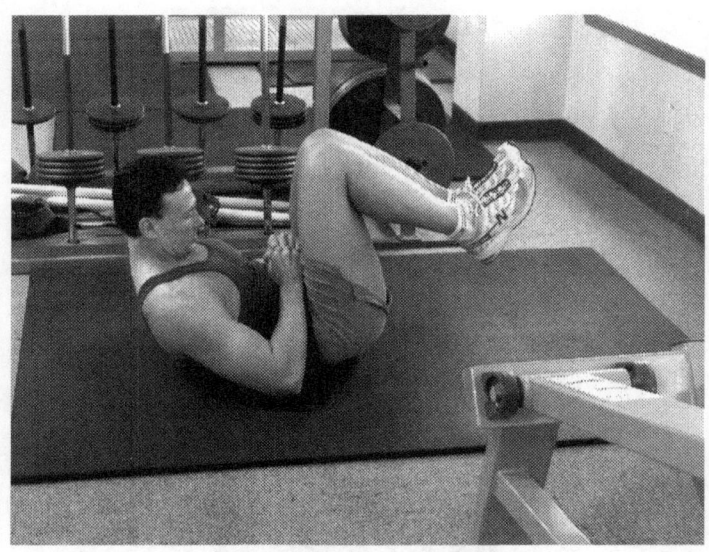

**Abdominals – Crunches (Finish)**

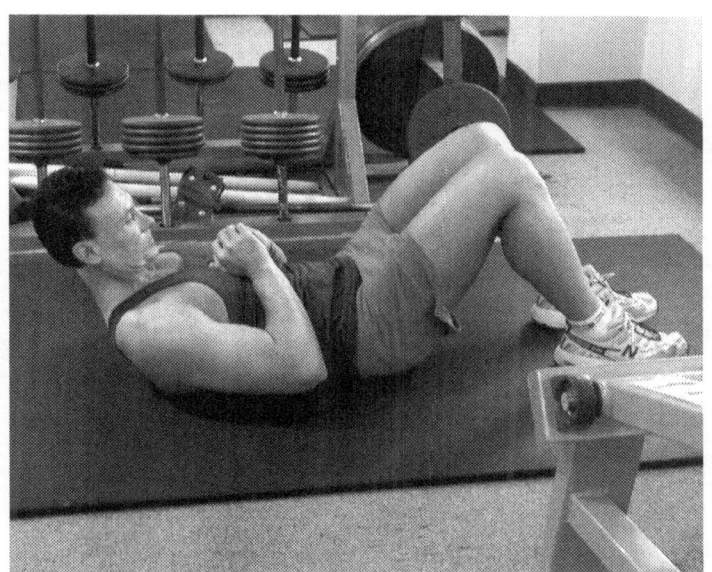

**Abdominals - Bent Knee Sit-ups (Start)**

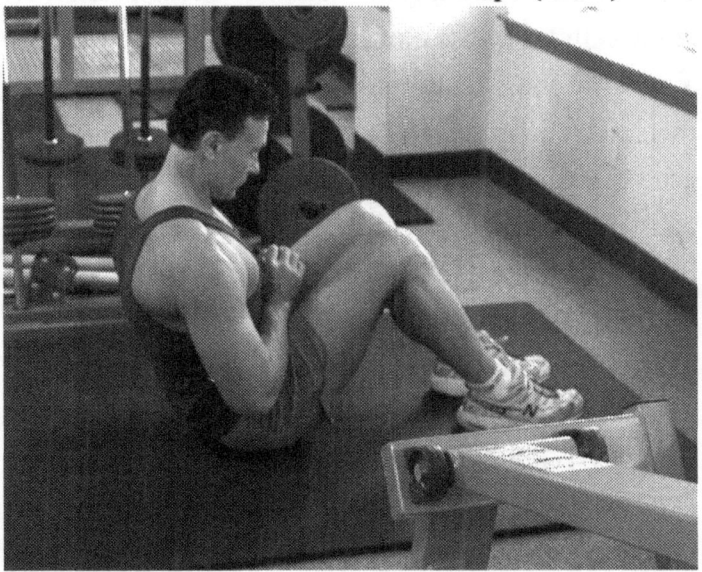

**Abdominals – Bent Knee Sit- Ups (Finish)**

## Catabolic vs. Anabolic
## An Exercise Myth Exposed

Though a fine line separates the two, your body is either in a state of consumption (breaking down) or construction (building up). In simple terms, your diet and exercise habits have a direct bearing on whether your body is tearing itself down (a catabolic state) or in a state of growth (an anabolic state). Remember that your body's need for nourishment is constant, so any decrease in calories over time, increase in activity, or even sleeping for eight hours, can put you in a catabolic state. If your consumption of proteins, carbohydrates, and fats are adequate enough for repair at the cellular level following exercise, you can sustain a state of consistent 'construction' of new tissue. In this 'anabolic' state, all the needs for maintenance and growth are met through nutrition, intervals of time, rest, and your ability to avoid destructive emotional states that cause stress and anxiety.

With the implementation of resistance training (weight training), you can and should put your body in an anabolic or 'growth' phase. This is accomplished in two ways. First, the amount of protein, carbohydrate, and fat calories you consume, and second, by the timing of when these calories are consumed. Skipping breakfast, as many of us do, after eight hours of sleep, breaks the consistency of constant nourishment and works to prevent a state of anabolic activity. You cannot skip meals, especially protein intake, if you wish to maintain this state, and, believe me, this is a good state to be in. Why? Because in this state you are either maintaining or increasing your muscle mass, and this mass keeps your engine 'hot', where your daily calorie burn is maximized with or without exercise. By the way, these results apply to both men and women.

When you begin aerobic activity or starve yourself, you convert to the catabolic state, and though this is not where you want to be most of the time, look a catabolism as a necessary evil for losing body fat. In the 'tearing down' phase, fat cells are eliminated, and that's a good thing. But other cells are consumed too, including some lean muscle tissue. It is virtually impossible not to lose some 'lean tissue' when you perform your aerobic activity. Losing or 'burning off' fat cells and lean tissue cells come with the territory, but if you are consuming enough protein before and after each exercise session, you can keep the destruction of lean tissue to a minimum.

When you exercise, you are intentionally inducing a state of catabolic or anabolic activity. Each workout should be designed specifically for one or the other, but not both. The only exception to this would be your beginning phase of exercise. If you are, in fact, a beginner, low intensity weight training (one set per muscle group), and low impact cardio (aerobic training, such as walking), can and should be combined in the same session. However, as you advance to moderate levels of training, I highly recommend separating aerobic (commonly called 'cardio') and strength training. If you induce a catabolic state through a thirty- minute treadmill session, following it with weight training will be counterproductive because you have reached the 'tearing down' phase that your body needs nourishment and time to recuperate from. The same is true in reverse. Don't follow an intense weight- training workout with a long -term aerobic session. Your goal is to intentionally put your body into one to these states, but not both, because they cannot exist simultaneously. It is important that you know this and intentionally separate the two activities. A fifteen- minute walk before weight training is acceptable, if it's done for the purpose of elevating your heart rate and breathing in preparation for training. Your pre workout and post workout meals are designed for the specific purpose of either providing you with more or less carbohydrates(fuel), depending on the activity. Remember, carbohydrates and proteins are needed for resistance training, and carbohydrates should be restricted before aerobic training for best results. Moving forward, you now know that aerobics and resistance training should not be combined in the same workout once you have reached advanced levels of exercise. It is important that you have a clear understanding of these 'states' so your mistakes will be few and your frustration levels can be minimized.

## Guidelines for Maximum Exercise Results

1. Before any aerobic activity, your meals should be mostly high-protein, low fat, and low carbohydrate. This will help to optimize the amount of fat burned while retaining your mass (muscle volume). In addition, waiting a few hours (Example: Two hours after a 500 calorie meal), will yield better results.

2. Before resistance training, high protein, high carbohydrate, and low fat meals are best. Building mass requires the fuel provided by carbohydrates. Make sure carbs and protein are included in your post-workout meal too.

3. Stay away from calorie rich, heavy foods before your workouts. High calorie, fatty foods require time, energy, and effort on the part of your digestive system. With high volumes of blood being used to aid in your digestion, it will detract from the volume of blood your muscles require during

exercise (Hence, feelings of nausea, dizziness, and cramps).

4.  When you feel tired or fatigued before your workout, cut back on the volume or length of your session, but try not to eliminate it. You should know when you are too fatigued and should not continue. Key point- if you are over-training, you may feel fatigued, irritable, and, because exercise stress effects your immune system, you may be vulnerable to colds and other health problems. Learn to identify the difference between over-training and one night's lack of sleep. If you feel tired for days at a time, give yourself a few days rest.

5.  For maximum results from weight training, change the order, pace, weight, and intensity (speed) of each workout regularly. Your body eventually adapts to the same sequence of exercises and your results will eventually level out. Change is good here. The shock of the new and different will have a much greater effect on your body and mind, eliminating that 'stale' feeling or the boredom of the same routine.

6.  Hydrate yourself before and after each training session by drinking water. If necessary, drink only small amounts of water (one to two ounces) during your workout. Keep in mind that working up a sweat

is fine, but too much sweating is counterproductive. Your muscles require the minerals and fluids that are lost when you sweat, so keep it to a minimum.

7. If you tend to be disorganized, keep a diary of both your daily summary of activity, and nutrition. Not much is needed to monitor each day. Summarize your efforts. Grade them using whatever scale you please, and refer back to previous days to take advantage of the habits or activities that gave you the best results in the past.

8. Allow your body the time it needs to recuperate from training. Growth and recovery occur between your workouts.

9. Keep it natural. No drugs. No alcohol. No stimulants. If you are a coffee drinker, try switching to tea. To insure a natural sleep cycle, stay away from stimulants in the evening.

10. Find a training partner that has your level of passion and fits the same general profile as you. For best results, train with someone that is slightly more advanced. It's great for motivation, but beware of dips and lapses in commitment levels from time to time. Remember, becoming co-dependent does nothing for your own internal drive.

11. Set a "Fat Loss" goal, not a weight loss goal. The scale can be inaccurate in determining results from

exercise and diet combined if you have gained some lean muscle. Learn to measure your own fat percentage level, either with your own caliper, or by someone who is qualified. For men, a healthy, attainable level (what Doctors have recommended) is 11-15%, for women, 19-23%. If you want that 'six pack' look for summer, you may have to set your sight on a goal that is much lower.

*Chapter 6*

## Nutrition 101

To provide you with a thorough understanding of nutritional needs, and for the purpose of simplicity, let's look at the breakdown of food into three categories. **Protein, Carbohydrates, and Fats.** All food groups, including meats, vegetables, cereals and grains, dairy products, and fruits are combinations of one, two, or all three of these categories.

**Protein.** This is the building block for both growth and maintenance. Not just for muscle, protein plays a role in almost all activities at the cellular level. When you exercise, your protein needs increase. If resistance training (weight training) is part of your program, your protein requirements increase even more. Protein rich foods, such as chicken, fish, eggs, pork, beef, and other meats, should be your primary food source. Protein is measured in grams, and the amount of grams you need daily can and will differ throughout your lifetime. Young, adult, active males may require well over 150 grams per day, whereas, an inactive older male may require only half that quantity. As a rule, men generally require more protein because they are larger and their engines are fuel injected with a mix of testosterone, the hormone that aids in building and maintaining muscle mass. To find out what your specific needs are, you have to monitor your intake of protein. As a fifty -year old active male who trains with weights three times a week, I like to take in about 140 grams per day, or roughly 80 percent of my weight (175 lbs.). You, on the other hand, must look at your sex, age, weight, muscle mass, and exercise habits to determine your own level of daily intake. Protein is good. Appreciate and understand it.

**Carbohydrates.** If you think of carbohydrates as fuel, you have it right. Be it simple sugars(fructose), whole grain breads, rice, pasta, cereal, or potatoes, wholesome, natural foods high in carbohydrates are good, whether they be complex or simple by nature. It's you that make them evil. Let's look at the car engine analogy again. We talked about the two things responsible for burning calories. Metabolism (involuntary) and Exercise (voluntary). Metabolism is your engine. If you exercise often, spread your meals to more than three per day, and carry more mass (muscle) on your frame than most, you may own a powerful, hot burning engine. If you are inactive, and spend most of each day starving yourself, your driving a small, mildly warm moped. Are you a Lamborghini, or a moped? Feeding your engine is the fuel tank. It should not always be full, but it should never be empty. You should have some general idea as to how active you will be from day to day, and you need to fill your tank accordingly. Short trips (lack of exercise) require less fuel. So if you have no choice but to sit on your ass for the next few days (your job requirement, for example), excess carbohydrate calories will be stored as new fat cells. Yummy!

**Fats.** For balance, a small percentage of your diet can and should be fats. Ten to fifteen percent is usually a good starting point. There are two types of fat you should be aware of. First, the saturated fats, which are found in meats and dairy products, are the bad fats. These fats contribute to poor health in the way of excess body fat, heart disease, and arterial damage. The good fats, the omega threes, and others that are typically found in both salt and freshwater fish and related seafood, can be either good for you, or harmless. Read food labels for fat content, and limit your saturated fat intake, as well as your 'fat calorie' intake. I understand that fatty foods tend to be very tasty. Remember what I said before about pace and limitations. It may work for you to take one day each week and indulge, as long as the other six days you can maintain that ten to fifteen percent range of fat intake.

## A Simple Plan

Your diet should consist predominantly of protein and carbohydrates, and little fat. I favor a 45/40/15 ratio (45% protein, 40% carbohydrates, 15% fats). This means 45 percent of my daily calorie intake is from protein, 40 percent from carbohydrates, and only 15 percent from fats. High protein ratios are necessary for anyone involved in resistance training several times per week. This is where you must do some experimenting with your own intake. Keep in mind that this is a guideline I developed according to my needs as a middle-aged, adult male involved in intense resistance training. If you have to keep a diary for a month, do it. Change your levels of proteins and carbohydrates to a level that fits your body and your exercise habits. Again, in a perfect world, you would decrease your carbohydrate intake throughout the day, taking in the smallest amounts in the evening, where it makes no sense to fuel a body that will be at rest for eight to twelve hours. If your goal is lowering your percentage of fat, beginning your aerobic activity on an empty stomach is the best plan. This means first thing in the morning, or a few hours after a meal. Before your body begins to use stored fat as a source for fuel, it will use the energy from existing carbohydrates(both simple and complex), so it makes sense to begin aerobic activity with as few available carbohydrates as possible. The more you load up on carbohydrates prior to your aerobic activity, the longer it will take your body to convert from 'energy burning' to 'fat burning'. Remember, your goal is to lower your percentage of body fat, not just to burn a lot of calories and make that 30 minute goal on the treadmill. Get my point? With resistance training, however, you should put some fuel in the tank.

Remember, carbohydrates are good and allow for maximum energy and strength during workouts or any other physical activity. If you are a beginner and have poor eating and exercise habits (you should know this by now), develop a simple strategy for eating. If you are a sugar lover, cut your consumption in half. Meat lovers - cut your consumption of saturated fats in half. You should have a clear understanding of your weaknesses with diet by now, and moving forward you will have no choice but to succeed if your attitude towards food relative to energy is a re-programmed part of your thinking. As I explained earlier, you need to work on eliminating your 'resistance' to your current faulty reasoning. Remember, most people you will know in your lifetime won't have anything to offer you on this subject because almost everyone in America needs some form of de-programming. If you challenge my point on this, you are being foolish, and if you choose to live in a state of ignorant denial like most, you always move laterally through life with everything you do, but never upward. So take the 'food as energy' philosophy to heart, keep things in balance, and keep your plan of action simple.

## The Importance of Water

Though water is found abundantly in the things we eat, no matter what the source, the importance of drinking water cannot be understated. The cells of your own body are mostly water. Water aids in metabolism and organ function, cleaning and providing vital nutrition to every cell. Many health problems can be linked directly to de-hydration (lack of water). The nutritional advice of eight glasses of water per day is sound. You should take heed, my friend. If you are not a 'water drinker', learn to become one. Drinking an eight- ounce glass of water before each meal is an excellent way to lower the volume of your meals, and allows for slow, methodical weight loss in a very healthy way. In fact, if I could only give you one piece of advice regarding diet and weight loss, it would be the implementation of more water in your diet. Not soft drinks, coffee, or milk - but water. When you exercise, water aids in cell growth and repair, and, depending on the duration and stress of your exercise regimen, your need for water will increase. The best habit you can begin to develop now is drinking more water. The second best habit is developing an exercise routine and seeing it through again and again, until it, too, becomes habit.

## The Good, The Bad, and the Worst Foods

Now comes the easy part of your journey. No more looking inside at your defects and working on your flawed programming. You, as a capable reader, should already have a working knowledge of nutrition. Protein, Carbohydrates, and fats can all be measured in calories. That dreaded calorie. I remember the good old days of dieting when all you had to do was carry around your little calorie counter booklet. A bit anal, but it helps to some degree. The mistake most of us make is that the source of your calories is just as important as the counting. Looking at the fuel analogy again, with the concept of you burning the calories you take in daily, there is a lot of burn involved in a raw carrot, versus, for example, a piece of cake. The best foods are natural whole grains, meats low in fat, and raw fruits and vegetables. Dairy products are usually part of the major food groups, too, but beware of the fat content. Once any food is canned, it usually loses nutritional value and falls into the 'processed' food category, which are marginally good at best. Foods that are good for you are simple. No additives. No preservatives. They usually require minimal cooking, if any, and they are rarely calorie rich. Try to keep your intake of saturated fats to a minimum by limiting dairy products, foods fried in vegetable oil, and meats high in fat. A steak or a hamburger won't hurt if it's broiled or low in fat content. Foods that are canned, boxed, frozen, or just wrapped in plastic can be good or bad. Look at volume and weight compared to calories, preservatives, fat content, processed sugars, sodium levels (salt), or other 'additives' not provided by nature.

## The Good

**Typical choices for healthy, daily nutrition:**

**Breakfast:**

**Egg White Omelet**- prepared in non-stick pan, ½ tablespoon of olive oil, with one yolk per 4 egg whites. Mix in an ounce of 99% fat free turkey bacon or sausage if you want a little more flavor.

**Oatmeal/Cream of Wheat/ Bran Cereal** - prepared in combination with berries or fruits and low-fat milk if desired. No sugar. Add sugar substitute, cinnamon, or any other spice desired for flavor.

**Other Suggestions** - Whole wheat toast(no butter or margarine), yogurt, whole grain bagels, bran muffins, fruit juice, vegetable juice.

**Lunch/Daily Meals**

**Broiled or grilled Chicken or Fish** -A great low fat source of protein. Add seasonings to taste and minimal salt.

**Tuna -** either broiled or out of the can (packed in water). Mix in a small amount of light mayonnaise (if desired), and mustard to taste.

**Salads -** any type of raw vegetable salad, maybe some pasta or beans, with low fat dressing.

**Vegetables -** Steamed or raw, preferably fresh or frozen, with very little butter, margarine, or salt.

**Fruits/Fruit Salads -** keep it fresh, without syrup or added sugar.

**Dinner/Evening Meals**

**Lean Sirloin Burger or Steak, grilled, or Fish/ Chicken -** ( Note the consistent high protein intake), steamed vegetables, preferably green, such as peas, green beans, or broccoli. Add a salad if desired.

Note that quantities are not mentioned. Adaptation of quantities will be determined by you, according to your own needs. Men and women will differ in protein, carbohydrate, and fat intake needs relative to size, age, and activity levels. Note too, that there should be a tapering off of carbohydrates at the end of each day, especially if you are resolved to very little activity in the evening. Personally, I like to indulge in red meat once or twice a week, and my off- days may include high fat content red meat, poultry, or even pork.

What are the worst foods? Well, the answers here are easy. But you will have to read food labels and contents descriptions, and you have to make wise, non-impulsive decisions about what foods to purchase. You will need to be diligent and become educated in your buying habits in order to recognize them. Foods high in fats, high in processed sugars, high in additives, and generally, any foods that are concentrated in calories in relation to size and weight, are bad for you. My rule of thumb on protein sources is the ratio of protein to fat grams. Generally speaking, if a packaged dinner contains 30 grams of protein and only 15 grams of fat, I consider it satisfactory. Ideally, you should try to consume only 3 grams of fat for every 10 grams of protein (33%) while you are in your 'strict diet' mode. Knowing the total calorie and carbohydrate counts of what you purchase are just as critical, as well as your knowledge of what 'trash' carbohydrates are. Remember, processed sugar (white sugar), corn syrup, processed flours and starches, and white bread or rice offer little nutritional value. If you choose the weekend to liberate yourself for culinary pleasure, try to keep your fat to protein ratio at least one to one and limit your consumption of trash carbohydrates. If eaten in moderation, some of these tasty foods will have little effect on you. My warning here is that of continuous consumption. Again, the philosophy of 'balance' comes into play too.

Eating properly is not rocket science, though many of us play the 'ignorant' game. Let's expose the dangerous, self-rationalizing internal voice we all have, and some of us (I'm not naming names) will make this statement to ourselves; "I have a poor diet because I don't know any better and nobody ever told me how to eat right." Sound familiar? Unless you live in a cave in Tibet, you **have** been given enough knowledge, and this knowledge has always been available to you. Sometimes it is our nature not to even put forth the effort, even when the knowledge of how to succeed is there. Why? What is it about our nature that holds us back? The answers are forthcoming.

## The Supplement World - Product Overload!?

If you are aware of the sheer number of products on the supplement market, you need to be educated on most of the diet and performance supplements that are available. Again, the same basic principle of consistent turnover and profit underscores most of the products being advertised. Not all of them are vital to your health and ability to lose weight, but some are quite effective and can work in conjunction with proper diet and exercise. The confusion in the marketplace lies in the quantity of vitamins, minerals, stimulants, appetite suppressants, and herbal remedies. As I mentioned earlier, I could care less about corporate America and the exaggerated claims. I rely on my own 'biofeedback' when testing the effectiveness of supplements, and you should too. Above all, your focus should always be on natural, organic vitamins, minerals, and herbs. Through thirty years of training experience, I have found that sticking to the basics is always the best and the least costly method. Indeed, if your diet has shaped up, and you maintain a balance of quality foods, your need for supplements is diminished. We do, however, live in a 'toxic' society, where the quality of food, our fast-paced, overstressed daily lives, and even the air we breathe can increase your need to supplement through the consumption of vitamins, minerals, and herbal remedies. Keeping things simple, I recommend a daily intake of a quality vitamin/mineral supplement. My personal favorites are those with high levels of minerals, B-complex (the B vitamins), and vitamin C. A good litmus test of quality is to check the label for the microgram content of B-12. Commonly known for it's positive effect on energy levels, B-12 is an expensive vitamin to produce, so a label with a high level (18 mcg or more) is a good indicator that the manufacturer didn't go the cheap route.

The current choices you have for stimulants and energy enhancement are overwhelming too. Again, results tend to differ from person to person, so some experimentation is needed on your part. Caffeine is the common choice of most Americans only because it permeates the beverage industry. Caffeine can be moderately productive if taken intentionally, preferably early in the day, and as a pre-workout stimulant. Other moderately successful herbs are Ginseng and Green Tea. Ginseng appears to improve stamina and sustain energy levels. Green Tea has re-gained its popularity recently in the enhancement of weight loss. Some of the claims behind its success are the lowering of cholesterol levels and the ability to inhibit the main enzymes involved in the storing of fat. What I suggest here is a small investment on your part. If any product out there can truly depress your appetite and not jeopardize your health in the process, I say try it. Remember, however, that more is not better, so keep your doses moderate. Stay away from anything that stimulates a few hours before bedtime, too.

Again, note that I seem to pound away at the recurring theme of balance and moderation. The supplement world is no different. Some of these compounds can be harmful, even lethal, if taken in high enough doses. There are also a few borderline 'natural' stimulants on the market that are almost in the drug classification. Keep in mind that the Food and Drug Administration has very little control over the supplement world. Claims can and will be over the top and recommended dosages may sometimes be in question. So play it smart, keep it natural, use what works for you, and do some research on your own. Your ability to think independently and not follow the 'latest and greatest' fad is at play here too.

## Chapter 7

### The Pain of Change

I have put forth some sound, fundamental questions about human behavior that needed to be answered, and, by now, you should begin to create a clear picture of your own behavior. Why are you overweight? What unknown entity restricts you from doing what you know to be positive most of the time? Why do we all tend to sabotage our efforts or become complacent in our attitudes? There are, after all, unexplainable fears that all humans have. One universal question I've always had about myself and the rest of mankind, is 'Why do we resist positive change'? A very valid question, indeed. Why do you eat too much and exercise too little? No one wants to feel miserable and out of shape. Why don't we overcome these irrational fears that prevent us from taking action? You and I deserve to know the answers.

My conclusion, and I am confident that you will agree, is that although these fears are 'phantom' in nature, they **do** exist in our minds. Fear is the most irrational, sabotaging emotion we all have. It's the driver of the car that controls our collective unconscious. What we must understand about our nature is that most fear is irrational. As I mentioned earlier, real danger rarely exists. We simply invent our fears as we go along. We resist change, even if it's good for us, simply because of this ever -present fear of the unknown. There is something very odd, but very true about our nature as humans. When confronted with someone or something that is unknown, our first impulse is to develop a negative mental image. In this case, the unknown is the image of a new, fit and trim, you. Fear of failure, or even fear of success, are part of the roadblock to your effort to achieve permanent weight loss. After all, if you never try, you can never fail, and your mistakes in life will be few. Nice and comfortable and risk free. Many of us live our lives this way. It's time to get out of your comfort zone and take some chances. You will have to force change in the beginning, and it will feel uncomfortable, but if you break through your 'fear barrier' intentionally, efforts in permanent weight loss will take hold as new habits. The question now is - 'Are you willing to push through your own false barriers'? If you can't expand out of this comfortable little zone you built around your psyche, you are doomed only to moderation in everything you do. Be fearless and do not be afraid to take risks with your efforts to change. Remember what I said earlier about control. Control applies here, too. Control, in combination with the confidence that you have conquered your fears, will lead you to many great endeavors, not just in the way of improving your diet, but in all areas of your life. You should never, I repeat, never fear positive change.

## Finally

I know what you wanted when you first started reading. More than likely it was a list of what to eat for breakfast, lunch, and dinner that will be the answer to all your prayers. The words will jump off the page, become engrained in your mind, and, from that moment in time forward, your transformation is on auto -pilot. Like being hypnotized, you just 'fall' in to a new lifestyle of discipline and attitude changes. Fact is, before you even picked up this book, you had healthy concepts of what to eat and how to exercise. You just never applied them before. This is the point in time where you decide to throw away your crutch. The choice you must make now involves the rest of your life and how you will choose to live it. Remember the rationale you used in the past. All lies you told yourself many times over. Can you look in the mirror and see what is really there? Do you understand that it truly is nobody's fault but yours? Stop the denial and blame games you play regarding control. You are in control, and you must face the music. Stop searching for the 'quick fix' diet or supplement and accept that the path will be long and steady, but extremely rewarding.

Now, let's get down to you, specifically. It's self-assessment time. Sit down and make a list of every reason you eat other than to sustain your life and your activities. Get off your ass and just walk if you must, but do something if you are sedentary and wish to begin. Yes, you are faced with a long journey, but a single step is all that is needed to start, and here's the non-sugar -coated part. If you don't, you will die before your time. Your quality of life from this point forward will be a fraction of what it could be. Realize that some people have no choice if they are handicapped physically or mentally. So why would you choose to treat your body so poorly and forgo any quality of life you would have in middle and old age? Like I said before, your health is the single most important commodity you own. All the wealth, power, and social status you

131

accumulate in your life up to this point is worthless if you jeopardize your health in the process. Know now that the internal rationale of "I'll start my diet tomorrow" or "I'll join a gym next week" is not only pathetic, but dangerous. Understand that perpetuating a lie, especially to yourself, is as bad as drug addiction in that it will eventually destroy your health. Begin to put some conscious effort into your health, and start to take control. Recognize and accept your weak points. You have no coach, no drill instructor, and probably very few people to emulate, so, of course, it's not going to be a cakewalk. At first. But remember, new efforts in discipline will eventually become habit, rejuvenate your soul, and give you a level of enjoyment you thought could never exist.

So what have you discovered? There is an underlying suggestion throughout this publication that information is deliberately being kept from you as a consumer. Do you understand what this information is? First and foremost, there is no such thing as 'instant' success in world of nutrition or fitness. Can you lose ten pounds in ten days? And, if so, how healthy would it be? You now know these answers and you should now know that your 'diet' will go far beyond the physical. Do you truly understand that the majority of Americans are misled? Do you understand just how important it is to question what has led us astray as a society? Let me clarify my point in them form of this question. Do you want to be one of those grandparents who is forced to only sit and watch as your grandchildren play, or one who participates with equal enthusiasm? If you follow the crowd, look outward for answers, and accept that a poor quality of life is your fate, then your life will be a fraction of what it can be. The next time you read a book or an article on weight loss, or even a suggested diet, you should be aware of just how much is left out of the equation. If you have gained just a little understanding of what is truly being pushed hard in the marketplace, you should see it clearly and even find humor in most of it now. You should now understand that though the majority may rule, the majority can mislead the few, and, in your case, you have the knowledge to put yourself in the righteous minority. To boil things down for you, the decision you now face is to accept or deny your former faulty beliefs, your faulty reasoning, and if you accept and admit there existence, you can change them. Once you break through this wall, you can begin to take action and start to conquer the unthinkable.

The power of your mind is virtually limitless. You can accomplish great things and still never reach your potential. Begin your journey by exercising your mind. Discover what makes you weak and strengthen it. A healthy diet and exercise mean nothing without understanding, control, discipline, and the effort to overcome your fears. The only way to break the cycle of continuous failed efforts is to discover **why** you eat too much or exercise too little. Develop your meditation and visualization skills. Develop a 'Loner' mentality. Stop seeking approval and place value on yourself for a change. If you are of an unselfish nature, a 'pleaser', you will need to take intentional, conscious, and even emotionally painful steps in order to become your own person. Once you begin to apply your new discipline, repetition and will power will evolve into an almost subconscious habit, and the strained effort of your early days will be forgotten because they have become second nature. It is critical that you understand this fact: **Losing weight permanently is a psychological process of evolution, with diet and exercise playing only minor, secondary roles.** Remember, you have one hundred hours each week to deal with your own impulses and you spend less than nine hours each week exercising and eating. So why hasn't anyone ever taught you and I how to successfully manage this interval time? Isn't the time between meals and exercising more critical? Few companies would be willing to market anything relative to psychology or "How to Manage Your Interval Time". I call it the 'Path of Least Resistance' in our open market. It's much easier to show people how to exercise and provide a grocery list of the foods to eat. Believe me, they haven't done you any favors. The message diet companies are sending you is "Look how much we can help you with those nine hours each week. Screw the other one hundred hours - you are on your own!" If you look strictly at the numbers, with instruction on diet and exercise consuming nine hours each week, but no instruction or suggestions on how to get through the other one hundred, you only have a nine percent chance of success! Are you beginning to understand the flawed way we view diet and exercise and that some of these engrained beliefs are perpetuated by your own ignorance? You should. Stop looking outward for direction on the other one hundred hours. They are yours and yours alone to manage. Substitution therapy, meditation, visualization, and identifying your own 'triggers' all come into play with those one hundred hours. I have given you the tools to help manage this interval time. But the catch, for you, is that they must be applied. You will have to get of your ass. You will have to do some soul-searching to find your own alternative passions and distractions. As I mentioned before, your roadblock of fear may have to be destroyed. If it is, in fact, overwhelming to you, or if you think you may need counseling, then seek it. Refer back to the five steps of empowerment I covered earlier and the concept of what truly is 'the perfect diet', and it will help you. Food is an addiction for some. Only a handful of weight loss counselors, authors of diet books, or even personal trainers are qualified to handle the mental de-programming it will take for each of us to be successful in our effort (again, information not commonly disclosed in the media). What I can tell you is that millions of people have accomplished this on their own before you and I came along. They did it without counseling or guidance from the latest 'fad' diets or weight loss centers. This is good news for you. Now that you know of others who have reached the top of the mountain, your journey should not be the psychological struggle you assumed it would be. Start to make a plan. Write it down. Post it in a place that forces you to confront your goals every day. Stop caring about ridicule from others when your behavior and attitudes differ from the 'mainstream'. Remember, the planning and physical follow through of what you want to achieve is the easy part. Never rely on external motivation. Rely on yourself. Work on your flawed thinking and habits as a project that will never be completed, but more importantly, enjoy the process because it can be very enjoyable. Overcoming your irrational fears and destructive thinking can and will be very liberating.

So go forth, my dieting friend, and enjoy your journey of discovery - revel in it, have fun with it, and apply what you learn about yourself. Once you begin to do this, a funny thing will happen. Your old, irrational, miserable, frustrating lifestyle will disappear. Good luck, good fortune, happiness, and boundless energy will find you. Once you get to this new place, reward yourself. The path has been laid out and the credit for success will belong to you and you alone. **My guarantee to you as a reader is that I will never take credit for what you accomplish, no matter how much you have relied on or put into practice the tools I have given you to be successful. In the end, there is only you and your own untapped, internal power.**

### Your 'To Do' List

1. Do something physical every day
2. Meditate and visualize your end results every day
3. Bring balance into your life
4. When in doubt, or confused, always refer back to the philosophy of 'The Perfect Diet'
5. Control and conquer your fear of change
6. Become an independent thinker (Develop a 'Loner' Mentality)
7. Leave your comfort zone intentionally(Overcome irrational fears)

8. Find and cultivate anything positive that distracts you from craving more food than you need (Substitution Therapy)
9. Never attempt to control what you are powerless to control
10. Become a student again. Take the initiative to learn about nutrition, exercise, and human behavior so you can identify your own 'triggers'
11. Always question the mass appeal of anything when financial gain is at stake
12. Set a goal, develop a plan, and learn to enjoy both the effort and the results

www.ingramcontent.com/pod-product-compliance
Lightning Source LLC
Chambersburg PA
CBHW061307280526
45784CB00002B/931